WEIGH LESS,
LIVE LONGER

WEIGH LESS, LIVE LONGER

Dr. Lou Aronne's "Getting Healthy" Plan for Permanent Weight Control

Louis J. Aronne, M.D.

with Fred Graver

A ROBERT L. BERNSTEIN BOOK

John Wiley & Sons, Inc.

New York · Chichester · Weinheim · Toronto · Singapore · Brisbane

Copyright © 1996 by Louis J. Aronne, M.D., and Fred Graver
Published by John Wiley & Sons, Inc.

First Wiley mass market edition published 1997.

The information contained in this book is not intended to serve as a replacement for the advice of a physician. Any use of the information set forth in this book is at the reader's discretion. The author and publisher specifically disclaim any and all liability arising directly from the use or application of any information contained in this book. A health care professional should be consulted prior to following any new diet.

ISBN 0-471-58112-7
       0-471-17695-8 (mass market)

Printed in the United States of America

10 9 8 7 6 5 4 3 2

I would like to dedicate this book to my many patients who have taught me so much about this disorder. Their willpower and struggle to succeed, even in the face of enormous challenges, has made my work even more worthwhile.

ACKNOWLEDGMENTS

First, I would like to thank my wife, Jane, and children, Allison and Louis, for putting up with me and the many things I do that take me away from them. In addition, my parents Theresa and Albert, my sister Adrienne, and Zack, Patty, Andrea, Frank, and Warren, Uncles Andy and Frank, and Aunts Lucille and Ann provided invaluable inspiration. Without their support, this book would not have been possible.

This book is a synthesis of many ideas and concepts. Some of them are my own, and some have been adapted from the colleagues with whom I practice and conduct research. I would like to thank them all, but in particular the major contributors:

Jules Hirsch, M.D., allowed me to join his lab at Rockefeller University. As he predicted, what I learned there radically changed my views about obesity and its causes. Rudy Leibel, M.D., generously shared his data and vast fund of knowledge about obesity and metabolism. The scientific sections of this book owe much to his guidance and willingness to review the manuscript. Ron Mackintosh, Ph.D., helped me stay focused on our research throughout this period. Michael Rosenbaum, M.D., Streamson Chua, M.D., Ph.D., and the other members of the lab have always been helpful, as has Karen Segal, Ph.D., at Cornell.

Janet Feinstein, M.S., R.D., designed and calculated all of the diets and recipes in the book. Kathy Isoldi, M.S., R.D., reviewed the diets and gave other helpful advice. The insightful contributions of Deborah Levitt, Ph.D., on psychology provide the foundation for the information here. Richard Weil, M.Ed., put together the exercise program based on his work with diabetic and high-risk overweight patients and showed that anyone can exercise.

Fred Graver, my co-author, got the book going despite his many other commitments, and I am grateful for the enormous enthusiasm and energy he devoted to the project.

Karyn Feiden extensively edited this book, making it more accessible and readable than I could have hoped for. She got the book finished, no small task given the hectic nature of my life.

My thanks to Bob Bernstein, who encouraged me to start this book, PJ Dempsey, senior editor at John Wiley and Sons, who helped guide me through the whole editorial process, and all of the other people at John Wiley, including Carole Hall, DeeDee DeBartlo, John Cook, Mary Dorian, and Chris Jackson.

Rich LaRocco of the Cornell University Department of Medical Art and Photography drew all of the illustrations efficiently, on time, and within budget.

My assistant, Darshna Parekh, helped me with absolutely everything.

Thanks also to Gayle Gardner, my co-host on the *Getting Healthy* program at the Television Food Network, and to Mauri Small, our producer, and Kim Greenberg, our assistant producer. Their ongoing support has helped our cable television program to thrive.

My sincere thanks to William R. Berkley, Herbert Siegel, and Michael Steinhardt, for their wise advice and generous ongoing support for our research projects.

CONTENTS

❖

PART THREE
THE NUTS AND BOLTS OF DIETING

PART FOUR
TWO MENU PLANS THAT WORK

PART FIVE
THE EXERCISE PROGRAM

INTRODUCTION

———————— ◆ ————————

Before we begin walking together down the path toward good health and weight control, there are two things you should know about me: First, I'm not a "diet doctor"—I am a doctor of internal medicine. Although I head New York Hospital's Weight Control Center, I am concerned, first and foremost, about the overall health of the people I treat. But the clinical research I conduct at Cornell University Medical College and at Rockefeller University, combined with the many people I see in my practice, has helped me understand the close links between illness and weight. When I look for ways to help ailing people, I often find that shedding excess pounds is the best place to begin.

The second important piece of information I want to share with you is that I am not very thin. I'm not overweight, but I'm hardly competing for the cover of the fashion magazines. I am, on the other hand, very healthy. I watch what I eat, practice the nutritional principles described here, and exercise regularly. I have a relaxed and positive relationship with food, and I enjoy healthy, satisfying, and regular meals.

My attitude reflects my philosophy. I'm not interested in being as thin as a fashion model. That's not my body type, and very likely it isn't yours either. Despite the myths perpetuated in

1

the fashion industry and the media, I don't believe there is any such thing as an ideal weight that is right for everyone. We've all got different metabolisms, different bone structures, and different dietary habits. But we *can* all reach a place that allows us to feel comfortable with our bodies and content with how and what we eat.

Over the years, I have made a number of major lifestyle changes. When I was growing up in the 1950s and 1960s, I ate a diet familiar to many Americans, at least those of Italian descent. There was meat on the table at almost every meal—pork chops, lamb chops, steak, chicken, pasta with meatballs. Fresh vegetables were a rarity. Legumes, such as peas and beans, were viewed as something served by people who couldn't afford anything better.

My food habits outside the home were even worse. When I was a child, my mother would telephone a restaurant in advance so that an order of spare ribs was on the table when I arrived. As a teenager, I worked at the local sweet shop, where I was allowed to help myself to ice-cream sundaes drenched with syrup and whipped cream.

This steady diet of meats and sugars, combined with my genetic makeup, gave me a tendency to gain weight. It seemed as if I was destined to follow in my family's footsteps. All of my relatives had gotten heavier as they got older and most of them had paid a high price for their excess weight. My enormous grandfather died of a heart attack at fifty-two. My grandmother, who described herself as weighing "two pounds less than a horse," died of breast cancer.

By the time I got to college I was, to put it politely, rather portly. When I decided to join the lacrosse team, I realized it was time to get serious about losing some weight. I opted for drastic measures. I went on a rigid high-protein diet, and within a week I had shed 15 pounds. But I felt terrible. I could not concentrate on my schoolwork and my body ached ferociously. I decided that if I had to deprive myself of so much pleasure in order to get thin, I would just remain fat my whole life. Within a few weeks, I had gained back all the weight I had lost.

My knowledge of weight control became more sophisticated when I began studying medicine at Johns Hopkins University in Baltimore. I had the good fortune to share an apartment with a student from China who introduced me to an entirely different way of eating. He prepared attractive meals of well-seasoned rice and vegetables, sometimes flavored with modest amounts of chicken and fish. The tastes were so delicious and satisfying that I stopped craving old favorites, like pastrami, corned beef, Italian hero sandwiches, and deep-fried dishes. During the year we lived together, I lost 25 pounds with very little conscious effort.

That weight loss changed my life. I looked great, or so my friends told me, but more importantly, I felt terrific. I was more active, more energetic, and better able to concentrate on my tasks than I had been in years. Inspired by my own experience, I began studying the relationship between weight and health. Back then, in the late 1970s and early 1980s, there were a few classic academic papers published on weight control and fat cells, but ongoing research was poorly funded and the subject attracted little scientific attention. Most of what we now know about weight gain was only idle speculation, and few physicians were focused on finding better ways to treat overweight people.

After completing my residency and fellowship, I joined the faculty at New York Hospital/Cornell Medical Center in 1986. As an internist, I was soon treating people with a host of chronic ailments, including diabetes, high blood pressure, arthritis, and coronary disease. Most of them were substantially overweight and seemed to be adding pounds with every passing year. Weight was obviously the primary cause of their medical problems, and it was frustrating to treat their symptoms without addressing the underlying cause.

Within a year, I had made one of the most important decisions of my career. I approached R. Gordon Douglas, M.D., then the chief of medicine at Cornell, and proposed a comprehensive weight control and health-care program. I got the green light, and by 1986, the Weight Control Center was up and running. We brought nutritionists, exercise physiologists, and a psychologist on board in order to address the many dimensions of weight control comprehensively. And soon we began to see some clear results. Initially, we used a liquid diet, but over time we developed a more flexible, food-based approach that worked for many people. By following our diet plan, sticking with an exercise regimen, and making some significant changes in their eating habits, our clients were losing weight. More importantly, they were keeping the weight off and their health was improving.

In the years since I became involved in the field of weight control, there have been enormous scientific strides. The link between weight and health has become a fertile area of research and is widely recognized as a crucial component of good medical care. In one of the breakthrough findings of the decade, laboratory researchers have been able to identify several of the genes associated with obesity in animal models. And in the summer of 1995, a series of landmark studies described the role of leptin, a hormone that apparently plays a central role in weight regulation by reporting body fat levels to the brain. The original research, conducted with mice, suggested that genetic programming results in the production of a mutated leptin molecule. In humans, obesity seems more likely to be a result of a weak brain response to leptin's effects. Although treatments based on these findings won't be available immediately, they support the theory that some people are cursed with the tendency to gain weight easily.

We have also learned more about the role that metabolism and brain chemistry play in weight control and have begun to understand so-called *weight set points* and the compensating mechanism called the *reduced state*, which is probably the result of increased muscle efficiency and makes it so hard to maintain lost weight. We also understand more about the psychology of eating disorders and have a more sophisticated explanation for the ways in which exercise can prevent people from regaining lost weight.

Thousands of people have been treated at the New York Hospital/Cornell Medical Center, and many of them have learned to win at weight control. I'd like to share their approach with you. This book provides comprehensive medical advice and weight control guidelines pulled together from my clinical practice and my experiences as a member of the Laboratory of Human Behavior and Metabolism at Rockefeller University. It also draws heavily on the cutting-edge work many of my friends and colleagues do in the fields of weight control, psychology, nutrition, and exercise physiology.

I'm living proof that the principles I'll be sharing with you in this book really do work. Given my family history, I view this as a small triumph. I have lost my taste for heavy foods, and I have learned to exercise. I have kept the weight off during the prime weight-gaining years of thirty to forty-five, and my last cholesterol count was an impressively low 165. Most important of all, I have stayed healthy, and medical research suggests that I have drastically reduced my chances of becoming ill in the future.

PART ONE

THE SCIENCE
OF
WEIGHT CONTROL

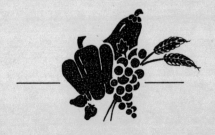

❖ ❖ ❖

1

INTRODUCING THE GETTING HEALTHY APPROACH

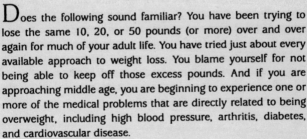

Does the following sound familiar? You have been trying to lose the same 10, 20, or 50 pounds (or more) over and over again for much of your adult life. You have tried just about every available approach to weight loss. You blame yourself for not being able to keep off those excess pounds. And if you are approaching middle age, you are beginning to experience one or more of the medical problems that are directly related to being overweight, including high blood pressure, arthritis, diabetes, and cardiovascular disease.

You are not alone. Excess weight is the number one nutritional problem in the United States today. Ten years ago, one-quarter of the American population was clinically obese, defined as a weight that is 20 percent or more than desirable. Today, that figure has leaped to 33 percent. We don't yet have an easy fix for this problem, but we are making major strides.

Weigh Less, Live Longer is not like other diet books you may have used. I offer no easy formulas for weight loss, no magic bullet that will melt the pounds away. I'm much more concerned about how you feel than how you look. And I'm convinced that a single set of rules is not suitable for everyone who is trying to lose weight.

Most people are initially motivated to diet because they want to improve their appearance. I guarantee that's going to happen when you reach a healthy weight, but there are limits to how thin you can be. You are only setting yourself up for failure if you try to push your body further than it is designed to go. The Getting Healthy approach focuses, first and foremost, on avoiding the preventable medical problems associated with being overweight—good looks naturally follow.

This book has ambitious goals. I want to teach you how to design a weight control program that will last for a lifetime. My role is to give you the best and most current information available, but I'm counting on you to participate actively in your dieting decisions. I'll supply you with menu plans and recipes that you can follow to the letter, but I am also going to make it easy for you to improvise. I'll give you all the information you need to undertake this program by yourself, but if you want some additional guidance from a physician, dietitian, or professional counselor, I'll tell you how to find someone who will be supportive.

Although medication can sometimes be helpful, the best, longest-lasting way to gain control over your weight right now is through your own efforts. I'm here to point the way, but you are the one who must make the journey.

THE REVOLUTION IN WEIGHT CONTROL

This is probably the most exciting time in history for the field of weight control. A combination of research and clinical experience has led to an explosion of knowledge. A revolution is taking place in the way doctors think about overweight people. Obesity is finally being recognized as a chronic medical condition that needs a medical solution.

We now know that the traditional goal of dieting—to reach

some fashion magazine concept of an ideal body weight—is impossible for most people. Weight is as individualized as height, pulse rate, or blood pressure. We never ask people to become taller or shorter. We don't blame them for having asthma or a skin rash. And it is just as illogical to ask people to become thinner than their bodies allow.

We have also learned that it is possible to change your metabolism and to teach your body to burn more calories. This is a long, slow process, but it works. To alter your body's physiology, you have to eat differently and exercise a lot more. You also have to discard some habits that may have become familiar enough to feel like old friends. None of this is easy to do, but if you can manage it, you can stop the endless and frustrating cycle of dieting, gaining weight, and dieting again.

Our new knowledge allows us to completely rethink the way we've been treating weight problems. The traditional culprits, such as overeating and laziness, are much less relevant than we ever thought possible. Instead of blaming you for being fat, we can now concentrate on helping you live a healthy life and win the struggle against your natural tendency to put on pounds. The Getting Healthy approach brings together all the latest techniques to help you lose pounds slowly, sensibly, and permanently.

"What's Wrong with Me?"

Here are some clues that your current approach to eating and weight control isn't working for you:

- ❖ You add a few more pounds to your weight every year.
- ❖ You cycle through a pattern of dieting, giving up, and dieting again.
- ❖ You lose weight, but it returns within a few months.

Many overweight people who seek professional help from me have reached the end of their rope. They have used every new diet on the market yet the weight keeps coming back, usually with a few extra pounds added to every gain-loss-gain cycle. They have starved themselves, given up sweets and starches, and constructed elaborate systems of punishments and rewards as motivational tools.

But nothing has worked. They feel frustrated, guilty, and burdened by self-doubt. Over and over again they tell me: "I just don't understand what I'm doing wrong."

The first thing I say to anyone trying to diet is this: "It's not your fault that you are overweight. The origins of your problem lie mostly in the genes you have inherited and the habits you have acquired over a lifetime."

But then I emphasize something else: "You are not helpless. Far from it. It is your responsibility to learn how your body works, to understand the eating patterns that contribute to weight gain, and to make some changes."

When I begin to work with someone new, I usually emphasize the importance of having the right attitude toward dieting. If you are like most of the people I work with, you may have failed so often that when you begin a new diet, you expect to fail again.

I see things differently. I know how hard you have been trying. I believe in you and I am going to help you learn to believe in yourself. I suspect you have been poorly served by some of the myths that abound in our society—namely, that thinner is always better and that there is a miracle cure for your weight problem.

If you are willing to work with me, if you are open to some new ideas about food and are ready to make some changes in your lifestyle, we can make some real progress. With perseverance, you will be able to stop thinking of food as your enemy and start developing a flexible, common-sense, and realistic relationship to it. You can give up drastic diets, stop wondering if you are going to fit into your clothes, and begin to enjoy the simple pleasures of eating. Best of all, you can start heading down the road to good health and a fine-looking body.

THE SOLUTION IS IN YOUR HANDS

One thing that often gets in the way of making a commitment to weight control is the feeling that you are being forced to adhere to someone else's ideas. That's not what the Getting Healthy experience is all about.

I see my role as an architect and educator—I can give you the blueprint you need to build a weight control program and teach you how to use it, but ultimately you are the one who has to construct the plan. Your personality has a definite impact on the type of weight control program that will work for you. For example:

❖ Do you function best when you are given a lot of structure? Or do you thrive on uncertainty and risk taking?
  Your answer will suggest how rigid your menu plans should be.

❖ Are you the type of individual who thrives under pressure? Or do you prefer a slower pace of life?
  Your answer will influence the exercise regimen you use.

❖ Do you like to surround yourself with close friends and family members? Or do you perform best when you are left alone?
  Your answer will help you decide whether to ask someone else for support.

In this book, we talk a lot about why people gain weight so that you are in a better position to understand what you can do about it. Here is what you can expect to learn:

  ❖ Why some foods make you fatter than others
  ❖ What to do about food cravings
  ❖ How your body gains and loses weight
  ❖ How your body processes food and stores fat
  ❖ How you can break unhealthy eating patterns
  ❖ How you can train your body to burn more calories
  ❖ How to maintain weight loss

❖ How to shop and prepare foods the Getting Healthy way
❖ How to control weight for a lifetime

In the long run, people who lose weight successfully—and keep it off—become skilled problem solvers. The ones who do best with my program are willing to look frankly at their own situation, gather a body of comprehensive information, and then make their own choices. They are realistic about themselves and they understand how to build on their strengths and plan for their weaknesses. They have their facts straight about fats and calories and know that reducing slowly is the only approach that works.

One of my patients religiously followed the nutritional principles explained in this book—six days a week. On the seventh day, he would indulge himself at dinnertime. Sometimes that meant taking his children to a fast-food restaurant; at other times it meant eating a favorite dessert. Knowing that he could splurge once a week gave him something to anticipate and prevented him from feeling deprived. The program worked well for him and he was able to meet his weight-loss goals without much difficulty.

THE THREE-STEP APPROACH: DIET, EXERCISE, AND BEHAVIORIAL CHANGE

A great deal of attention has been paid to the idea that diets aren't effective. The truth is not so simple. Conventional diets work for the job they were designed to do—in the short term, you can shed pounds by restricting the number of calories you consume.

But the lost weight won't stay off. Dieting can't be a way of life. There are very few people who can adhere to a strict diet for more than a few months. If you don't change your behavior, your body's natural tendency to replace lost weight always kicks in, and when it does, you'll find yourself heavier and less healthy than ever. To win the struggle against weight permanently, you have to work with your body, not fight against it.

No matter what your genetic makeup, you need to control these three factors in order to lose weight and keep it off:

Diet   Eating sensibly and sanely is one of the best ways to improve your health. The Getting Healthy menu plans are based on sound nutritional principles and are designed to achieve gradual weight loss so that you never feel deprived. By teaching you to eat right from the start, there is no need ever to go on a maintenance program. The Getting Healthy approach *is* a maintenance program. Two diet plans and a number of recipes are presented in Part Four. As you develop confidence in your ability to lose weight, you can also use my system of food exchanges and substitutions.

I usually urge my patients to begin with Menu Plan I, which is a low-fat, high-carbohydrate approach. If you haven't lost about a pound every two weeks over two months, I recommend switching to Menu Plan II, which is known as the lower glycemic index approach. This plan is based on recent knowledge about insulin resistance and minimizes foods that cause a significant rise in blood sugar levels, such as most simple carbohydrates and starches, while emphasizing fibrous vegetables, which have only a modest impact. With either plan, you'll be counting your calories carefully because you can have a perfectly balanced, low-fat diet and still gain weight if you consume too much food. Contrary to a myth that has become popular these days, calories *do* make a difference!

Exercise   The only way to maintain weight loss is to exercise on a regular basis. If you are accustomed to a sedentary life, I'll show you how to begin slowly and to build up your stamina gradually. Even if your fitness level allows you to walk just a few minutes a day, I am very strict about the need to get moving. The boost you get from exercise burns some calories right away, but more importantly, it greatly improves your body's long-term ability to maintain a lower weight. The exercises described in Part V will also help you tone specific parts of your body. Although spot reducing (trying to lose weight in a specific part of the body) doesn't work, it is possible to increase the amount of muscle on your body. And the more muscle you have, the healthier you will look.

Behavioral Changes   Developing smart food habits and changing behaviors that interfere with weight loss are crucial parts of my program. Some people just need to shop more intelligently, cook more healthfully, and eat more slowly. Others need to take a hard look at themselves and explore the stresses that may trigger overeating. Several chapters help you establish healthy habits. I also show you how to keep a weight control journal where you can define your goals, measure your progress, and identify any obstacles you encounter.

Some people give equal attention to diet, exercise, and behavior. Others may need to make the biggest changes in one particular area. For example, one woman I work with eats nutritionally sound foods, but she doesn't exercise and her habits are terrible: She eats just one big meal late in the evening after starving herself all day, so she ends up gaining weight. I emphasize the importance of all three components. Sure, you might eat too much on one particular day. Another day you might get no exercise at all. But if you are staging a three-pronged attack, chances are successes in one realm will cancel out a little carelessness somewhere else.

GETTING HEALTHY FOODS

Let's admit it: Eating is fun. I certainly enjoy my meals. Once in a while I crave bacon and eggs for breakfast. I've even been known to order a hot dog and french fries. But my weight is set to a reasonably healthy level, and I know that indulging occasionally won't have too much impact on my weight, as long as I quickly return to my usual healthy eating patterns.

When your weight is under control and you're working effectively with your body, you too will be able to splurge now and then. Right now, it is best to postpone indulgences. But take heart—once you have lost some weight and kept it off for a reasonable period of time, you'll have a lot more guilt-free opportunities to eat the foods you love.

A central principle of the Getting Healthy approach is that you should eat less meat and more fruits, vegetables, grains, and legumes. We are not suggesting that you stop eating meat altogether, but most Americans need to cut way back. I'm going to show you how to do that without feeling deprived. Once you understand some basic nutritional and cooking principles and start experimenting, there are an infinite number of opportunities to prepare low-fat, high-flavor meals.

Ever hear of quinoa? It is pronounced *keen-wah*, and it is a scrumptious, easy-to-cook grain favored by the Peruvian Indians because it is so high in protein. You might also try couscous, a light and flavorful grain popular in the Middle East. Fragrant rices from India, such as basmati and jasmine, are also readily available in many parts of the country. Many health-food stores sell these products in bulk, but you can also buy them in quick-cook packages that come with seasonings, cooking instructions, and recipes.

The point is that healthy eating doesn't have to be dull. Far from it. When you learn to use fresh herbs, lemon, and a full complement of spices from around the world, your food will be richly flavored and delicious, as well as nutritious. Chances are you'll never be able to go back to fatty foods and heavy meat dishes again.

CHANGING ATTITUDES ABOUT WEIGHT

Along with helping you learn to control your weight, I've written this book for another important reason—I hope it will help change the negative attitudes we have toward overweight people in this country. This troubling form of prejudice has not received much attention, but people who carry extra pounds on their body clearly face discrimination at work and in the community. They are misunderstood by their friends and families and often made to feel awkward, even unwelcome, in social settings.

The national obsession with weight results in the marketing of costly diet products that don't work. Forty billion dollars a year is being wasted on treatments for obesity while the connections between weight and health continue to be largely neglected. Meanwhile, the nation's health bill is soaring.

What can we do to erase this bigotry? How can we focus our limited resources more appropriately? I believe we need a national research and education effort focused on the realities of weight control, an equivalent of the President's Council on Physical Fitness. Former Surgeon General C. Everett Koop has made a noble start in this direction with his "Shape-Up America" project, and I'm convinced it would greatly improve the nation's fiscal and physical health—if Americans will give it a try.

These are the goals I would like to see emphasized in any national fitness effort:

❖ Help people understand that obesity is a complex medical problem.

❖ Educate people about the causes of obesity.

❖ Emphasize the links between health and weight.

❖ Combat discrimination against overweight people.

❖ Advance the science of weight control.

❖ Learn more about the techniques of weight-related behavior modification.

Fortunately, attitudes are beginning to change. There is a movement afoot to educate people and reduce the use of fad dieting. Groups like the National Association to Advance Fat Acceptance are talking about the mistreatment of overweight people. The medical community is beginning to recognize that obesity and eating disorders are medical conditions and that people who are afflicted deserve to be treated with understanding and respect. I'm delighted to see these enlightened perspectives emerge and proud to be playing a part in shaping this new way of thinking. I hope these attitudes will make us a healthier nation and create a better life for people with a weight problem and those who love them.

LET'S GET STARTED

Some experts believe it is almost impossible to change dietary habits. I disagree. It is a difficult task, but if you are determined and committed, it can be done. I've seen it happen over and over again.

If you follow the principles in this book, you will take a huge step toward a healthier, saner life. If you can master the tools you need for a lifetime of weight control, this will truly be the last diet book you'll ever need.

Congratulate yourself on having the courage and discipline to face the challenges ahead. Enjoy the sense of control you are about to gain. Start thinking about how good you are going to look and feel.

Let's get started.

2

UNDERSTANDING YOUR BODY

❖

How much food do you think you consume in a lifetime? The diagram of a truck, developed by Jules Hirsch, M.D., physician-in-chief and obesity researcher at the Rockefeller University Hospital, offers a startling visual clue.

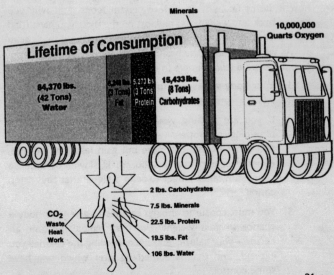

Lifetime of Consumption

Minerals

10,000,000 Quarts Oxygen

84,370 lbs. (42 Tons) Water

5,248 lbs. (3 Tons) Fat

5,273 lbs. (3 Tons) Protein

15,433 lbs. (8 Tons) Carbohydrates

2 lbs. Carbohydrates
7.5 lbs. Minerals
22.5 lbs. Protein
19.5 lbs. Fat
106 lbs. Water

CO_2
Waste
Heat
Work

Thin or fat, all human beings consume an enormous amount of food and water. Whether you gain excess weight as a result is, to a significant degree, a function of your genes and your metabolism. When we talk about making diet and lifestyle changes, we are really talking about what you can do to make your metabolism a partner, rather than an opponent, in your weight control efforts.

A number of interrelated factors—notably genetics, metabolism, and brain chemistry—conspire against your determination to lose weight. Does this mean that you have no control over your appetite? Not necessarily. Just who is in command here? You are. But only if you recognize the powerful forces that help to determine how much you eat and what you weigh.

Understanding, accepting, and mastering your body's natural tendency to gain weight spell the difference between winning and losing at weight control. Your problem is probably not a failure of willpower. You don't need a more drastic diet. What you do need is a better understanding of how your body works—how it stores fat, why you crave certain foods, and why you gained back any weight you had lost on the diets you have tried before. That is knowledge that can put you into the driver's seat.

As we run through the basic science relevant to weight control, there are a few pointers to remember:

1. Your body wants you to consume calories and to store fat.

2. If you are gaining weight, it is because you have a physiological propensity to do so. The nagging feeling that other people eat more but gain less may be true, either because your metabolism is slower or because your brain takes longer to send a signal that says "stop eating."

3. You must consume enough calories to give your body a chance to gain weight. Don't let biology become an excuse—your caloric intake is exceeding the calories you expend, and that is something over which you have some control.

4. To continue gaining weight, you have to be relatively inactive. The flip side: A program of regular exercise is a must if you are going to lose weight.

THE STORY OF EVOLUTION

The hunters and gatherers of early society lived on a roller coaster of feast and famine. When food was plentiful, they ate well. When the food ran out, they lived off the fat their bodies had stored during bountiful seasons. During times of famine, anyone who had not been able to store fat perished. Those who survived were those who were blessed with "fat-storing" genes that they passed on to subsequent generations.

This is the miracle of evolution, and we see the same characteristics in animals around the world. The dominant animal within most packs is the fat one. In Yellowstone National Park, for example, the fat bison are the only ones who survive the long winter. Some of us in the field of weight control like to say that Charles Darwin was a trifle off the mark: The great biologist and evolutionary theorist wrote that the *fittest* members of a species survive. We're beginning to realize that historically it has been the *fattest* ones who endured.

Descendants of early "fat-storing" people walk the earth today. But the modern Western diet has turned a desirable characteristic—the ability to survive by storing fat—into a major public health problem.

A compelling study of fat-storing genes and their impact on society was conducted by Eric Ravussin, Ph.D., and Clifford Bogardus, M.D., obesity researchers working for the National Institutes of Health in Arizona. Ravussin and Bogardus studied two groups of Pima Indians—one living on an Arizona reservation, the other in the remote Sierra Madre mountains of Mexico—and found remarkable differences between them. More than 80 percent of the Arizona Indians weighed twice the national average and most suffered from a host of medical complications as a result. Half of the study group had diabetes and 60 percent had gallbladder disease.

But in the primitive environment of the Mexican mountains, the Indians had only a 10-percent incidence of obesity and suffered very few of the diseases of their Westernized relatives. What these tribal cousins share are a similar genetic background that predisposes them to obesity and diabetes. But their daily patterns of life differ dramatically. Whereas the Arizona tribe no longer experiences food shortages, the Mexican Pimas continue to endure cycles of deprivation. For them, the primitive fat-storing capacity remains a lifesaving tool.

That distinction echoes throughout our society. In twentieth-century America, most of us are well fed and lucky enough to be able to secure food on a daily basis. Our ability to grow sufficient crops, and to distribute them efficiently, is a marvel that is unprecedented in history.

But our bodies are still genetically programmed to survive the feast-famine cycle. As a result, we keep storing calories, but never draw down our account. When we add in all the labor-saving devices that have greatly reduced our physical activity, it becomes apparent why the cycle of weight gain–loss–gain has changed to weight gain–gain–gain.

GENES, HORMONES, AND OBESITY

The struggle to convince physicians and scientists that the tendency to put on weight is rooted in biological structure has taken a dramatic step forward since scientists began isolating incriminating genes in animal models. The discovery of genetic mutations and hormonal deficiencies that cause obesity in animals received worldwide attention and lent credibility to the notion that human obesity may also have a genetic basis.

The notion that the ability to gain weight is inherited had been hypothesized for many years, supported in part by studies of identical twins, who gained excess weight in exactly the same way, in the same amounts, and in the same places on their bodies, even when they were raised in different homes. In the same studies, other twins raised apart stayed thin even when their food habits were very different.

Other early hints came from scientific studies of rodents with various genetic mutations that resulted in a condition that greatly resembles human obesity. When these rodents were fed the same diet as normal animals in the same family, the first group mushroomed to twice the size of the second group. This was viewed as further evidence that a genetic characteristic could be at work.

My colleague Rudolph Leibel, M.D., and his associates at Rockefeller University, are pioneers in this field. They spent several years inbreeding mice and searching for genetic clues to explain the differences between normal mice and their very obese siblings. Eventually, genetic tests were developed that allowed these researchers to predict from birth which animals were destined to become obese.

In the December 1994 issue of *Nature*, the specific mutation that causes the increased appetite and decreased metabolism of an obese mouse was reported by Yi Ying Zhang and her colleagues at Rockefeller University. We believe that if a mutant *ob* gene is present, the animal may not know whether or not it has stored enough fat to satisfy its current needs. Without the usual signal, the animal does not feel full, so it naturally keeps right on eating. The mutation may also explain why the animal's metabolic rate is slower than it should be.

More recently, Dr. Jose Caro, chief of medicine at Thomas Jefferson University School of Medicine in Philadelphia, and a group of other researchers at the same institution, published the sequence of an equivalent gene in obese humans (*Journal of Clinical Investigation*, June 1995). Interestingly, they did not find a mutation but did discover that the quantity of a hormone-like protein being produced was much greater than in normal-weight individuals. For some reason, the brains of overweight people may not receive the protein message properly—either because the message is blocked from the brain or because the brain response to the muscle and other organs is weaker than in normal-weight individuals.

In the summer of 1995, researchers went a step further when they isolated the fat-signaling hormone, now known as leptin, and clarified its role in weight control. Although published studies have been conducted only in mice, human beings manufacture an almost-identical hormone, stirring optimism about pharmaceutical treatments for obesity in the not-too-distant future.

Here is what we know so far: The fat cells of mice secrete leptin into the bloodstream. By monitoring those secretions, the brain determines how much fat is present. If hormonal levels are low, the mouse manufactures extra fat to compensate. If a substantial amount of leptin is present, the mouse tries to shed weight. The goal in both cases is to maintain a constant level of leptin, which increases as more fat is produced. In some obese mice, an inactive version of leptin is produced, resulting in massive weight gain regardless of food consumption. Even mice who produce normal leptin and gain weight by overeating lose weight when leptin is administered.

The exciting next step is to find out if human beings will respond equally well to leptin therapy. As this avenue of research is pursued, overweight people can feel more assured than ever that they are suffering from a metabolic disorder that deserves medical respect.

Recent discoveries are big steps along the road to finding better treatments to combat obesity, but there is still a long road ahead. It will be some time before scientists develop a drug to mimic the biological functions that may be disordered in some obese people, although pharmaceutical companies expect to launch human trials of injectable leptin very soon. There are medical precedents for the theory behind these trials—for example, insulin is routinely given to people with diabetes to lower blood sugar. Nonetheless, it is likely to be some time before effective treatment becomes widely available, and even when pharmaceutical options improve, they will complete, rather than substitute for, a rational program of diet and exercise. Don't let these exciting discoveries become an excuse for ignoring weight control now.

UNDERSTANDING METABOLISM

Metabolism is defined as the physical and chemical reactions that make it possible for your body to perform its basic daily functions. Your blood pressure, heart rate, and temperature are controlled by your metabolism and each of these functions has a *set point*: 98.6°F (37°C) is your temperature set point, for example.

Your body also seems to have a set point for weight and works hard to maintain it. Unfortunately, that point isn't always set at the right notch for optimal health. Just as high blood pressure or a fast heartbeat can cause medical problems, a high weight set point, or one that is poorly controlled, can lead to obesity and, all too often, associated ailments, if enough food is available.

A Theory about the Set Point

When you begin to overeat, the excess calories initially cause a small weight gain. Then, in an effort to maintain your set point, your metabolism speeds up to process the excess calories, your appetite decreases, and some of the newly gained weight drops off. We'll call this *metabolic resistance*.

From my clinical experience, I've developed a theory about resistance that makes sense to me, although I hasten to add that it is not yet proven fact. I suspect that in people with a chronic weight problem, the body puts up only a modest resistance to weight gain. On the other hand, people who do not gain weight readily may have more aggressive metabolic resistance.

If I'm right, your body may be quick to stop fighting its new weight. If you keep eating more calories than you burn, your metabolic resistance will quickly plateau and you will establish a new set point. With your weight stabilized at this higher level, it then becomes more difficult to lose those extra pounds.

We've got a lot to learn about why things seem to happen this way. It may be that new fat cells are produced or your brain may adapt to the new, higher weight. Whatever the biological explanation, the result is the same. Worse, the cycle of overeating followed by metabolic resistance, adaptation, and then weight gain can repeat itself endlessly in some people. Fifteen pounds becomes 30, then 50. At each point, the body readjusts its set point, so that during the resistance phase it is fighting to bring your weight down to the new set point, not the old one.

How the Set Point May Climb

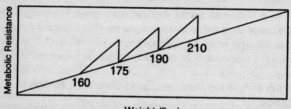

Weight (lbs.)

The Reduced State

A similar process occurs in reverse when you eat too little. Initially, your body slows down, burning fewer calories in an effort to keep your weight at the same level. That's why diets can be counterproductive: The harder you push your body to lose weight, the more forcefully it will work to keep the weight on. Cutting calorie intake too drastically results in very inefficient dieting—you won't lose as many pounds proportionate to the number of calories you stop consuming.

When you diet, you raise a warning flag that says famine is here. As a survival instinct, your body slows its metabolic rate well below the level needed to maintain your weight set point. Your metabolism is so shaken by the prospect of hunger that it slows way down to a *reduced state*.

The body never stops fighting weight loss. The metabolic mechanism is not fully understood but may be linked to an increased efficiency of muscle activity. Let's look at Mary Lou, who is 5 feet, 7 inches, and weighs 210 pounds. Five years ago, she weighed 160 pounds and needed 2,500 calories a day to maintain her weight. Now, at 210 pounds, she needs 2,800 calories a day. What would happen if Mary Lou suddenly cut her calories back to 2,500? Would her weight drop to 160 pounds? No. As she reduces caloric intake and loses weight, her metabolic rate slows and she will only drop to about 197 pounds, although she may be consuming the same number of calories as another woman of the same height who has maintained a steady weight of 160 pounds.

Mary Lou, like any dieter, encounters the reduced state when trying to lose weight. Like all of us, she will find it impossible to eliminate metabolic resistance to weight loss altogether, but a slow, steady approach to dieting helps minimize it.

UNDERSTANDING BRAIN CHEMISTRY

Controlling your weight would be a lot easier if it weren't for gnawing feelings of hunger. These feelings, and many of the other physiological and emotional states you associate with food, are triggered by chemicals inside the weight-regulating control center known as the hypothalamus.

The Hypothalamus: Your Hunger Center

The hypothalamus is the region of the brain that serves as the nerve control center for many metabolic functions crucial to appetite control. It sends out powerful chemical messengers, known as neurotransmitters, telling you when to eat, how much to eat, and even what to eat. Let's take a simplified look at the workings of a body in balance.

When the hypothalamus senses that you need energy—after you wake up in the morning, for example—it sends a messenger to tell the body to eat. One of these messengers is called neuropeptide Y (NPY) and its message is, "eat carbohydrates." This surge of NPY is experienced as hunger. NPY wants fast energy and it is equally satisfied with a piece of fruit or a cheese Danish.

Once the hypothalamus senses that you've eaten enough carbohydrates, it sends out serotonin to curb your appetite. Serotonin tells the body: "Slow down on the carbohydrates; you've had enough."

It sounds simple—some neurotransmitters say "eat"; some say "stop." But a number of things could go wrong in this delicate balance, for example, when:

❖ You eat a severely restricted diet.

❖ You are under stress.

❖ You are taking medications that affect your brain chemistry.

❖ Your metabolism is too slow for the appetite level set by your brain.

The Impact of Dieting

Some researchers believe that sweet cravings occur because there is too little serotonin in the hypothalamus. Without the appropriate information from the brain, you have no way to know that you should curb your appetite. By commanding you to eat sweets, your brain may be trying to raise its serotonin levels. One piece of evidence for this theory is that medication that raises serotonin levels seems to cut the appetite for sweets.

Cravings are also a common response to skipping meals or severely limiting your caloric intake. When the hypothalamus senses famine, it produces extra NPY to encourage you to eat carbohydrates. If you try to ignore that signal, the hypothalamus adds another chemical, galanin, to the brew. Galanin's message to your body is simple: "Eat fat. Store fat." Eventually, these messages become too insistent to resist.

Your brain chemistry can also be adversely affected by poor eating habits. If you try to satisfy the message to "eat carbohydrates" with simple sugar, the level of the hormone insulin in your bloodstream can jump, and your glucose level can peak and then drop sharply within a few hours. To protect you from plunging glucose levels, your body releases hormones that have the side effect of making you feel shaky and weak. Your immediate impulse is to find food—fast. The result is that you are riding a chemical roller coaster.

The Role of Stress

High levels of stress, such as those associated with family, work, or money problems, can also cause chemical imbalances in your body. Cortisol, typically produced by the adrenal glands when you are under pressure, tells your body to produce more NPY and may indirectly slow your metabolic rate way down. Stress also produces increased levels of galanin. As a result, you develop a craving for carbohydrates and fats.

To satisfy the powerful urge, you may indulge in high-fat, high-sugar foods, such as ice cream and chocolate-chip cookies, which trigger the production of serotonin and may stimulate opiate receptors. Serotonin has a drug-like, sedating, antidepressant effect on most people. As a result, eating actually may reduce stress. One of the biggest obstacles to weight control is that many people in high-stress situations effectively use food to medicate themselves.

HOW MUCH FAT CAN YOU STORE?

As if all of these genetic and metabolic challenges were not enough, someone committed to weight loss also has to grapple with the body's almost-endless capacity to store fat. Women are especially likely to store fat to protect the body's reproductive abilities. When estrogen levels soar at puberty, the body begins to produce high levels of galanin, as though it were trying to make sure you consume and save sufficient fat to help ensure the survival of the species.

Three independent factors affect fat storage:

1. How many fat cells you have
2. How large the fat cells are
3. Where excess calories are distributed

Think of a fat cell as a small balloon that can expand to three times its size. As fat cells fill with stored calories, they become larger and larger until they can hold no more and new cells are created. In general, people who are slender have the fewest fat cells of the smallest size. People who are modestly overweight may have equally few fat cells, but they tend to be larger than average. And obese people tend to have both more fat cells and bigger ones.

How Many Fat Cells You Have   Everyone has the capacity to keep producing fat cells but some people may do so much more readily than others. The average newborn comes equipped with a little more than one pound of fat cells and steadily produces more throughout childhood. Typically, these cells stop multiplying in adolescence, but the process may continue into adulthood.

The more fat cells you have, the more likely you are to store fat. And once fat cells are created, they are never lost. You can shrink your fat cells and lose some of the fat stored inside, but you can't lose the cells themselves. There they remain, eager to be filled again.

How Large Your Fat Cells Are   The size of your fat cells is one of the factors limiting how much weight you can lose. Fat cells are always at least partially full—the minimum size of a fat cell is about 30 percent of its size when filled with calories. Worse, your body has a tendency to resist cell shrinkage. If theories about the action of leptin are correct, you may get a chemical message that encourages you to eat more and slows your metabolic rate whenever your fat cells begin to contract.

Where Excess Calories Are Stored   What happens to the calories you eat? Some of them are burned immediately, as part of the digestive process, but excess calories of fat or carbohydrates float through the bloodstream and are drawn either to fat or muscle cells by the lipoprotein lipase (LPL) enzyme once the carbohydrate stores in the liver are full. LPL acts as a "welcome mat" on the cell. People who maintain a normal weight tend to send extra calories to the muscles, where they are burned, producing heat. Some people who are overweight may send a higher percentage of their calories to fat cells, where they are more likely to be stored.

The more LPL present on the cell surface, the more calories get drawn inside. The average person has three LPL molecules on fat cells to every one LPL molecule lodged on muscle cells, allowing three times as many calories to be stored as fat than muscle. And a number of metabolic factors, including high insulin levels, can increase LPLs on the fat cells, giving some people a fat-to-muscle ratio that is 4:1, 5:1, or even higher. According to a study by Robert Eckel, M.D., an obesity researcher and professor of medicine at the University of Colorado, dieting can actually increase the level of LPL on the fat cells whereas exercise increases the presence of the enzyme on the muscle cells. Obviously, that is one reason why exercise is such an important part of my program.

Insulin Resistance

Another biological mechanism that is highly individualized is insulin production. Insulin is a powerful hormone that drives blood sugar into cells and stimulates the liver to convert calories into their storable form. Historically, insulin helped assure the necessary reserves to survive famine. A current theory, however, holds that sugars and starches that are easily broken down in the intestines of most people raise blood sugar to excessive levels in some people. The pancreas then produces insulin in order to drive this excess sugar into fat and muscle cells.

In the insulin-resistant population, the cells eventually become inured to insulin's effects and the body is forced to produce increasingly larger amounts of the hormone in order to maintain normal blood sugar levels. The resulting high insulin levels in these people may be associated with numerous medical complications, including diabetes, high blood triglycerides, hypertension, and coronary artery diseases. They may also stimulate the appetite and lower the amount of sugar that is burned as energy while increasing the fat stores.

Genetics and environment both play important roles in insulin resistance. Some people are clearly predisposed to insulin resistance, but cigarette smoking, aging, obesity (especially in the abdominal region), and a diet high in simple carbohydrates and

starches can all worsen the problem. Even a diet high in saturated fat may exacerbate insulin resistance. On the other hand,
consuming monounsaturated fats, such as olive or canola oil,
may have a tempering effect. Normal fasting insulin levels fall
between 3.5 and 17; in our lab, we consider fasting levels above
25 as a sign of insulin resistance.

Insulin resistance helps explain why a low-fat, high-carbohydrate diet doesn't work for everyone and why some overweight
people do better by eating foods with a lower glycemic index.
The glycemic index measures the extent to which a given food
causes blood sugar levels to rise. It is really a measure of how
rapidly you digest starchy foods, and it is influenced by many
factors: the physical composition of your food, the degree to
which it has been processed, how long it is cooked, its dietary
fiber content, the frequency of your meals, the amount of solu-
ble fiber in your normal diet, and the other foods you are consuming at the same time.

It has been estimated that about 25 percent of the population are insulin resistant and therefore more likely to lose weight
with the lower glycemic index approach. While some of those
people may simply eat fewer calories on this diet, one recent
study suggests that the lower glycemic index, per se, does the
trick. Generally, I recommend starting with a low-calorie, low-fat,
high-carbohydrate diet, and if you don't see results in your waistline, switching to a diet where the carbohydrates have less effect
on blood sugar. You'll find both approaches in Part Four.

CAN YOU FIGHT HUNGER?

Now that you know how much basic biology is involved in
weight loss and weight gain, you may be asking yourself: Can
I tough it out? Can I fight the surge of NPY, galanin, and other
chemical messengers urging me to eat? Only for a short time.
Anyone who has ever used a traditional diet knows the cranky
feelings precipitated by the struggle to ignore the body's powerful

cravings. Unless you find ways to curb the level of the messages, you are eventually going to overeat.

That's why slowly changing your eating and exercise habits is the only practical approach to weight control. On the distant medical horizon are intriguing treatments for brain chemistry disorders. We are studying drugs that can increase serotonin and block galanin. We are hopeful that administering leptin will decrease appetite and increase metabolic rate. Eventually, pharmaceuticals may become a much more important part of weight control. But for now, the best approach is to reduce what you eat slowly enough to burn calories at a maximum level and to store them at a minimum level. That is efficient dieting. And that's what the Getting Healthy approach shows you how to do.

3

THE LINK BETWEEN
WEIGHT AND HEALTH

❖

The diseases of old age begin to take root in the middle years of life. In your thirties and forties, you may become more sedentary. As an adult with a full plate of work and family responsibilities, you probably have less time to watch your diet closely or to be physically active. Your metabolism begins to slow down as you settle into more regular, and typically fuller, eating patterns. In these years, it is easy to become careless. After all, you may think you are still too young and vigorous to worry about chronic diseases or to think much about using weight control to extend your life.

The Framingham Study, the most definitive study ever conducted on risk factors for heart disease, suggests this unconcern is a mistake. For the past three decades, investigators have been monitoring more than 3,000 men and women living in Framingham, Massachusetts. A substantial body of data has been collected to support the theory that the pounds you put on between the ages of thirty and forty-five are associated with numerous health problems later in life.

Fortunately, these middle years are also the time when it is easiest, and most productive, to stop gaining weight and begin taking control of your health. If I can convey only one message to you in this book, it is this: Don't treat your weight and your health as if they are separate issues. Losing weight now and keeping it off for good are two of the best things you can do to maintain or improve your health.

APPLES AND PEARS:
HOW BODY SHAPE AFFECTS HEALTH

There is mounting evidence to suggest that where you carry your weight is very significant to health. As the years pass, you may begin to notice the image of a pot-bellied middle-ager reflecting back at you. Once, a big belly was viewed as a symbol of success, a sign that someone was prosperous enough to eat without restraint. Now we recognize the truth—that kind of weight is a clear indication of health problems to come.

Some people—affectionately known as "apples"—tend to carry their weight in a roll around their waist and abdomen. Others are "pears" with excess weight on their hips, thighs, and buttocks. Although there is a strong genetic component to weight distribution, men generally tend to be apples and women tend to be pears.

Apples are more at risk for developing weight-related medical problems than pears because the fat carried within the abdominal wall goes straight into the liver before being circulated to the muscles. Fat in the liver tends to make that organ resist the effects of insulin. As a result, your insulin level may rise, possibly leading to elevated blood pressure and setting the stage for diabetes, hypertension, and cardiovascular disease. Pear-shaped people have a better medical prognosis, but a greater weight-loss challenge, since fat stored in the thighs, hips, and buttocks is broken down much more slowly than abdominal fat.

We use a measurement called the waist-to-hip ratio to determine whether you are an apple or a pear. To avoid increasing the risk of medical complications, a woman's waist size should ideally be less than 80 percent of her hips; a man's waist should be less than 95 percent of his hip size. In a study conducted among almost 42,000 Iowa women, ages fifty to sixty-nine, death rates climbed as waist-to-hip ratio increased. Other research has found that a high waist-to-hip ratio is associated with a greater risk of heart attacks among young men. In general, the lower your waist-to-hip ratio, the healthier you are likely to be. In Chapter 7, I'll show you how to calculate your own waist-to-hip ratio.

Meanwhile, take heart because the initial weight loss recommended in the Getting Healthy program—no more than 10 percent of your total body weight—typically comes off the abdomen. Even if you are determined to lose more after that, it is nice to know how much good you are doing yourself just by getting started.

THE MEDICAL RISKS

Among the specific health problems often associated with excess weight are:

- ❖ Bone and joint problems
- ❖ Diabetes
- ❖ Sleep apnea
- ❖ Heart disease
- ❖ Gallbladder disease
- ❖ Liver disease
- ❖ Certain forms of cancer

You may be healthy now, but your excess weight is straining all of the body's systems, putting you at increased risk of one or more of these medical conditions later. Although weight control does not guarantee long life, it certainly improves the odds. If your regular doctor doesn't raise the subject of weight control, you should.

Remember, too, that while excess weight can trigger illness, illness can cause weight gain. One reason is that illness may force you to become less active. Also, weight gain can be a side effect of medication. Talk to your doctor if your weight gain seems to be associated with drug treatment; it may be possible to switch medicines.

Bone and Joint Problems

When you are overweight, you place a great deal of stress on your musculoskeletal system. The formula I use to calculate the excess pressure on your weight-bearing joints is to double the amount of weight you have gained as an adult. For example, if you have put on 30 pounds since your early twenties, you have added 30 × 2 pounds of pressure to your joints—that's 60 extra pounds. At some point, you may actually outstrip your body's ability to carry its weight around. The stress is felt most keenly in the knees, hips, and ankles, which may become inflamed with arthritis.

The sooner you reach your healthiest weight, the fewer years of damage you will do to your body. Physical activity is especially important to minimize bone and joint problems. My exercise program (see Part Five) is geared to people who have been sedentary, and the graduated program of workouts are specifically designed to prevent injury.

Diabetes

Diabetes is caused by the body's inability to regulate the level of sugar in the bloodstream and is closely associated with obesity. When too much blood sugar is present, the pancreas produces extra insulin to force excess sugar into fat and muscle cells. Eventually, the regulating mechanism may be unable to keep up with the body's demand for insulin and the pancreas stops functioning. Adult-onset diabetes is the result.

Diabetes requires close medical supervision and can be life-threatening. Early symptoms of adult-onset diabetes are a dry mouth, blurry vision, and frequent urination, but the long-term effects can be premature coronary disease, stroke, kidney failure, and blindness. The first treatment a doctor will recommend is dietary modification. In my practice, we try to limit calories, as well as consumption of highly processed starchy foods, in order to lower the glycemic index, which is a measure of how much a particular food raises blood sugar. We also encourage people to increase their consumption of vegetables and some fruits. Studies have shown that when you change your diet and consume fewer calories, you may be able to bring your blood-sugar level under control even before weight loss begins.

Sleep Apnea

Sleep apnea, which is caused when the upper respiratory tract becomes obstructed, is a common problem among overweight people, especially men. While you are sleeping, your body weight may put your lungs and breathing passages under so much pressure that you cannot draw sufficient oxygen. You may literally stop breathing momentarily before being jerked awake in a life-prolonging impulse for air. Some people with sleep apnea may awaken hundreds of times throughout the night without realizing it.

Loud snoring is the most common symptom of sleep apnea, but other, more severe, symptoms may eventually develop. Some people become so fatigued as a result of their interrupted sleep patterns that they literally fall asleep without warning during the day. In its most severe form, sleep apnea can cause irregular heart rhythms and, rarely, heart failure.

Heart Disease

Excess weight clearly increases two major risk factors for heart disease: high blood cholesterol and high blood pressure.

High Blood Cholesterol   Low-density lipoprotein (LDL) cholesterol—popularly known as the "bad" cholesterol—is a hard, waxy substance that can clog the walls of your arteries and eventually lead to coronary artery disease. The effects of LDL can sometimes be mitigated by high-density lipoprotein (HDL) cholesterol, the "good" scavenger that takes LDL cholesterol from the cells to the liver for processing and disposal. When your cholesterol levels are measured, you are given both a total cholesterol count and a ratio between total cholesterol and HDL count. We hope for a total cholesterol level below

200 milligrams/deciliter and a ratio of less than 4:1, preferably closer to 3.5:1. Triglycerides, another form of fat, are also measured and should be less than 200 mg/dl. Again, the lower the better.

If you are overweight, particularly if your weight has settled mostly in the apple area around your waist and abdomen, chances are your cholesterol count will be higher. There is persuasive scientific evidence that high-fat foods, especially those high in saturated fat, increase cholesterol levels. The link between dietary cholesterol, such as that contained in shellfish, and blood cholesterol is more controversial and not fully proven. It is probably a reasonable precaution to avoid high-cholesterol foods anyway, but don't be lulled into complacency by products that claim to be low in cholesterol—they may still be loaded with saturated fat.

A modest weight loss can lower cholesterol counts dramatically, reducing the risk of coronary disease in the process. Shedding just 5 to 8 percent of your total body weight in a one-year period is often all it takes. There are no guarantees, however—some people have a cholesterol level with a very tightly controlled set point that does not readily change.

High Blood Pressure   There are no symptoms of high blood pressure, but the condition can lead to heart disease and can be life-threatening. Sometimes, high blood pressure is caused by adrenaline, which your body may produce in an effort to increase your metabolic rate and resist further weight gain. If you continue to add pounds despite this natural resistance, the higher adrenaline levels will eventually result in a corresponding rise in blood pressure. When your metabolic resistance to weight gain drops as you reach a new set point, your blood pressure may also fall, but seldom to the level it had been before you began gaining weight. The tendency to retain fluids, which is common among overweight people, adds to high blood pressure problems by increasing the pressure on your veins and arteries.

Anyone with high blood pressure needs to be medically supervised. Be sure to talk to your physician about the Getting Healthy program or other approaches to dieting because most people can lower their blood pressure by losing 10 to 20 percent of their total body weight.

Liver Disease

About one-quarter of the people enrolled in my weight control program have abnormal levels of fat in the liver, a condition that has been called "foie gras" of humans. Excess fat can inflame the liver and may eventually lead to chronic hepatitis or cirrhosis. The solution should not be a surprise—weight loss is the best way to prevent this particular liver disease.

Gallbladder Disease

A number of studies have begun to uncover a direct relationship between excess weight and the incidence of gallstones. We don't know exactly why, but bile, which is discharged into the small intestine by the liver to aid in the absorption of fat, seems to be the source of the problem. Apparently something goes wrong with the secretion of some combination of bile's three major components—cholesterol, lecithins, and bile acids—that precipitates gallstone formation. In general, women, especially pregnant women, are at higher risk for gallstones than men; we believe this is associated with higher estrogen levels, although the nature of the link is not entirely clear.

There are technical reasons why losing weight temporarily increases the chances of forming gallstones. Our best estimate is that about 10 percent of people will develop gallstones, even on a well-balanced diet. However, the Getting Healthy menu plans include sufficient fat and protein to allow the gallbladder to contract properly, which minimizes your risk. Your doctor may also advise you to take aspirin or a prescription medication, ursodiol. Despite the short-term hazard, weight loss significantly lowers your overall risk of gallstones.

Cancer

Many researchers have explored the complex link between weight and cancer in depth. Although it remains a subject of intensive scientific scrutiny, we don't yet know whether it is weight itself, or the fat in most Americans' diets, that may heighten the cancer risk. We do know that an American Cancer Society study has shown that cancer mortality increases in people who are 40 percent or more above their optimal body weight. And we suspect that dietary changes may lower the incidence of many life-threatening diseases, including colorectal, prostate, ovarian, endometrial, breast, and cervical cancers.

No one knows for sure how little fat will really lower your risk of cancer or how much excess weight significantly heightens the danger. However, there is enough statistical evidence to suggest that reducing both your weight and the amount of fat you consume—in particular, saturated fat—can make a significant difference.

PART TWO

GETTING THE
SUPPORT
YOU NEED

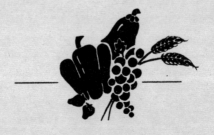

◆◆◆

4

THE EMOTIONAL
CHALLENGES

❖

Food and our relationship to it touches every area of our lives. Through food we express love and admit feelings of emptiness. We celebrate with food and use it as a drug to relieve anxiety. Food is the source of human health, yet we have seen that it can also lead to illness. For many of us, food is at once a source of pleasure and a cause of pain.

In American society, food is about much more than just fuel or nutrition. There are strong societal pressures to look good, and for women, at least, that means to look thin. There are also many deep-seated psychological issues and personal challenges that play a role in weight control. Some people may fear being thin because weight gives them a physical power, a way to wield their bodies as if they were weapons. Others hide within their bodies because they do not have enough confidence to handle attention from the opposite sex. Reduced self-esteem is a very common hallmark of overweight people.

By reducing slowly with the Getting Healthy program, you can gradually make the psychological adjustments to a thinner self. But first you need to understand how you may be using food as a psychological crutch. The goals of this chapter are to help you:

❖ Understand your relationship with food..

❖ Learn how women may internalize sexist messages that make them feel badly about themselves.

❖ Recognize the role that unresolved family issues often play in weight control.

❖ Understand the impact of negative thinking.

UNDERSTANDING YOUR RELATIONSHIP WITH FOOD

Leveling with yourself isn't easy. It means asking some tough questions about who you are, who and what is important to you, what you need, and how you go about getting it.

To begin the process of self-exploration, examine your use of food to determine if you are eating for reasons other than satisfying hunger. These questions might help:

❖ Do you often eat to cheer yourself up?

❖ Do you find that eating helps numb pain?

❖ Do you use food to avoid confronting problems?

❖ Are you always struggling to prevent weight gain with strict dieting, fasting, or excessively vigorous exercise?

❖ Do your concerns about body shape and weight dominate your self-image?

❖ Do you have recurrent episodes of binge eating in which you eat uncontrollably for a period of time?

❖ Do you sometimes feel that your eating binges won't ever stop?

❖ Do you ever deliberately induce vomiting or use diuretics or laxatives to purge yourself of food?

If you answered yes to even one of these questions, there is probably a psychological dimension to your weight problem.

You may be using food to ease your anxiety, cheer you up, or distract you from life's challenges. In the next chapter, we'll talk about counseling and other forms of support that may help you deal with the emotional baggage that interferes with a healthy attitude toward food.

An unlucky minority of people with weight problems have severe eating disorders, such as binging or bulimia. Binge eaters are people who can generally eat normally but from time to time lose control and consume excessive quantities of food. People who are bulimic binge or overeat and then may induce vomiting or take laxatives to purge themselves of the excess calories.

Scientific attempts to understand these disorders are in their infancy, but at least they are now recognized as legitimate medical conditions. As someone who has been watching the weight control field evolve for many years, I can tell you there is major progress. The standard psychiatric textbooks finally include formal classifications for binging and bulimia, and physicians have recognized that they need to be treated aggressively.

Sadly, a small but significant percentage of people who suffer from very severe eating disorders have been victims of some form of sexual or psychological abuse in the past. Many of these people use their weight as a shield from the world, disguising themselves and hiding their pain. Occasionally I encounter someone who is afraid to reach the weight held at the time an abuse occurred, fearing that it may cause the vulnerability to return. I almost always recommend that people who have been abused seek professional counseling to deal with these intensely painful experiences.

THE IMPACT OF SEXISM

A study of corporate chief executive offices around the country came to this startling conclusion: Most of the country's male business leaders are above-average weight yet most of their wives weigh less than the norm. This finding reveals much about the world of difference between men and women when it comes to weight control.

This finding tells us that society has a double standard for beauty. In many circles, it is considered acceptable for a man to sport a belly that hangs over his belt, but no one admires a woman who carries that kind of extra weight. The study also reminds us that every day, in hundreds of subtle ways, women learn that who they are is indistinguishable from what they weigh. The message is that to be fat is to be a failure; to be thin, a success.

This message has a powerful impact on a woman's self-image and how she feels about her own body. Many feminists have analyzed societal and personal attitudes toward food and I find their insights to be both provocative and useful. For example, in *Fat Is a Feminist Issue* (Berkley, 1994), author Susie Orbach explores the conflicting information women receive about food and fat in our society. She writes: "Women absorb a powerfully contradictory message vis-à-vis food and eating. It is good for others, but bad for the woman herself; healthy for others, harmful to the woman herself; full of love and nurturance for others, full of self-indulgence for herself."

The result of these sexist attitudes is that men tend to be more relaxed about losing weight than women. Typically, it takes some sort of dramatic event to force a man to confront a weight problem. In his forties, for example, he may discover that he has hypertension or high cholesterol. Or a friend may have a heart attack that serves as a wake-up call. Often men are also content with a limited weight loss. After dropping 10 to 20 percent of his original weight, a man may feel good enough about himself to stop dieting.

Women, on the other hand, tend to be more feverishly determined to lose weight, and they are much more impatient with their progress. They may follow the Getting Healthy recommendations to lose 10 percent of their body weight, but then resist my suggestion to take a break and let their bodies adjust. I also have a hard time persuading women that they need only to lose enough weight to improve their health. The message that thin is beautiful is so powerful that even after reaching a healthy weight, most women are still driven to shed more pounds.

Understanding Family Issues

Another psychological issue of great significance is the complex and powerful impact of family relationships. I have noticed that many people are slow to recognize this. For example, I was treating a woman who overate every time she attended a family get-together, and typically for several weeks afterward. Deborah Levitt, Ph.D., the psychologist in my office, reviewed her meticulous food diary and pointed out this connection. The insight was startling and inspired her to confront the longstanding, but largely ignored, link and to change her food habits.

Weight problems are especially common among people who grew up in households that were somewhat dysfunctional. If shared meals were a time of tension in your childhood, eating may stimulate an unconscious memory of a difficult past and the resulting anxiety can cause you to overeat. Even in happy homes, attitudes toward food can create weight problems. For example, if food was a sign of togetherness, eating may be the way that you comfort yourself with memories of your youth.

If most people in your family were overweight, chances are that life in your childhood home revolved around food. Food may have been the path your parents chose to express their love, offering it to you as a source of reassurance or as a reward for good behavior. No matter how well-meaning their intentions, the result is a widespread weight problem.

The psychological issues may be different if you are overweight but most people in your family are thin. It is common to feel a sense of inadequacy or shame when you compare your own body to the bodies of others in your family. There may be times when you feel that your family would love you more if you were thinner, which can make you feel guilty or depressed. Rather than losing weight to gain their love, you may stage an unconscious rebellion by sabotaging your dieting efforts.

When you try to take control of your relationship with food, you may encounter resistance from family members. Your mother may think you are rejecting long-respected traditions. Your father may think you are trying to distance yourself from the family. Other relatives may feel that your decision to lose weight reflects negatively on them. Finding ways to deal with these attitudes and assure family members that your diet is not a backhanded way of criticizing them is part of successful weight control.

UNDERSTANDING THE IMPACT OF NEGATIVE THINKING

Winning at weight control means feeling good about yourself— regardless of the sexist messages you may have internalized, regardless of the difficult childhood you may have experienced. To look good and to get healthy, you have to emerge from the shadows of a difficult past and strengthen your sense of self-esteem in the present.

Central to that task is to stop saying bad things about yourself. David D. Burns, M.D., a psychiatrist at the University of Pennsylvania's School of Medicine and the author of two insightful books on depression, *The Feeling Good Handbook* (New American Library/Dutton, 1990) and *Feeling Good: The New Mood Therapy* (Avon, 1992), has helped me understand how damaging internal messages can be. I have adapted his list of ten self-destructive messages to weight control. If you are sending yourself any of these messages, you may be unwittingly erecting a barrier to your efforts to lose weight.

Ten Messages That Can Ruin Your Weight Control Plan

1. **"I'm on the diet or off the diet."** You see weight control in black-and-white terms. If you do not adhere to your diet, even in small ways, you tell yourself that you have been a total failure. You might say: "I never should have eaten that cookie. I might just as well abandon my diet right now."

2. **"I blew it with one piece of cake."** You blow a single event (such as a lapse in your diet, a pound gained, or a

casual comment about your weight) out of proportion, linking it to a never-ending pattern of defeat. A typical message might be: "I ate too many sweets today. That proves that my diets always fail."

3. **"Everything is about my weight."** You allow every event in your life to be colored by your weight problem. The message you send says: "I weigh too much. I'll never find a partner or get a good job."

4. **"It's never enough."** When things go well—you lose a pound, you exercise vigorously, or you say "no" to temptation—you shrug it off as unimportant. Success never feels as real to you as failure. Typically, you may say: "Okay, I stayed on my diet this week. But that won't last; it never does."

5. **"Diets don't work for me."** You expect disaster even before the facts are in. No one can convince you that things might turn out well. Before getting on the scale, you might say, "I doubt I lost even a pound." If someone tells you about a new recipe, you say, "I doubt I will like it as much as the goodies I used to be able to eat."

6. **"I can't do it."** You exaggerate your own mistakes and build up other people's successes. Thinking that everyone else is more disciplined, more methodical, and more accomplished makes it easier for you to give up altogether. Exaggerators say things like, "Patricia has a great body and loves lifting weights. I'll never be able to work out like that."

7. **"I don't feel like dieting."** You allow yourself to be ruled by your feelings, even when you know that you are not being logical. Your attitude is, "If I feel it, it must be true." This becomes a good reason not to accomplish your weight control objectives. By saying, "There must have been a reason I ate that piece of cake," you can explain away your lapses of discipline.

8. **"I'm guilty."** In order to take any action, you first need to push your guilt button. You punish yourself for being

fat, telling yourself you must do something, and then sending a message saying you are a bad person because you did not do it. The essence of your message is: "I'm going to flog myself into dieting."

9. **"I'm a fat person."** Instead of seeing yourself as an individual, you describe yourself with a label. Rather than saying, "I'm talented and creative, but I do have a weight problem," you say, "I'm fat" or "I'm a failure."

10. **"It's not my fault."** On a subconscious level, you may try to convince yourself that your weight problem is the result of forces beyond your control. That gives you an easy excuse to do nothing about it. Although I do not think it is your fault, for the moment it has to be your responsibility.

Silencing Destructive Messages

Before you can silence any of those internal voices, you have to admit you are listening to them. Your grim perspective is distorting how you see the world. Then, you have to explain the psychological origins of your discontent. Finally, you have to stop all that negative thinking and start strengthening your sense of self-esteem. Only when you have put your psychological house in order will you be able to:

◆ Stop punishing yourself.

◆ Accept your limitations.

◆ Appreciate your strengths.

◆ Understand where food fits in your life.

◆ Replace your food obsession with a more constructive focus.

◆ Start thinking rationally about what you eat.

◆ Feel good about who you are.

You may need help to accomplish these goals. The next chapter talks about sources of support.

5

A HELPING HAND

Controlling your weight can be a lonely and difficult job. Many people initially experience dieting as a time of deprivation. Although I have tried to make the Getting Healthy approach as friendly and flexible as possible, there will still be many occasions when you must tell yourself, "No, I can't eat as much as I would like." Often, you will also be saying "no" to other people: "No, I can't join you for dessert." "No, I don't want to eat out because I am not yet confident enough about my new habits." Until you start a weight control plan, you may not realize how much of your social and professional life revolves around food.

Many people are initially able to draw on their own internal resources for support. Deep inside all of us lies a wellspring of determination and discipline that can be tapped in times of need. But at some point in the course of dieting, almost everyone begins to feel immensely frustrated. Often, people say to me, "I can't do this anymore! I give up. I'll never be thin."

I understand those feelings, and when they occur, I recommend that you look for help. There is no reason to endure the challenge of dieting alone. Finding someone who can give you some support—one person who believes in you and is committed to your success—can make all the difference in your struggle against weight. Many people say that working with someone else makes dieting easier and more fun.

You may want to choose a close friend, co-worker, family member, or spouse—anyone who will support you with encouraging words, offer you creative recipes, and perhaps even exercise with you. Or, you may want to turn to professionals. A talented physician, dietitian, or professional counselor can encourage you to stick with the Getting Healthy program and help you modify my guidelines in ways that work for you. There are also a number of commercial weight-loss programs to consider; unfortunately, most of them do not have very impressive track records.

I know that it can be very hard to ask for help. Many people with weight control problems have been criticized all their lives for being overweight. Asking for help may feel like another admission of wrongdoing or failure. Be careful about who you approach, aware that not everyone will understand your fears or respect your sensitivities. At this vulnerable time in your life, you deserve help from someone who will ease the pressures on you, not add to them.

FINDING A PERSONAL HELPER

If you want to ask a friend or a family member for support, first think carefully about your needs. Are you looking for someone who knows how to select healthy foods from a restaurant menu? A companion who will resist the buttered popcorn when you go to the movies together? Someone to spend the evening in your home until your urge to devour a pint of ice cream has passed? You may want someone who knows how to steer you back on course when you begin to lose focus and encourage you when you become frustrated. In social and business settings, you may be looking for an ally who can help deflect the pressure to eat unhealthy foods.

Make sure that your helper understands the extent of your needs. Weight control involves a lifetime commitment. Obviously, you can't ask someone to be available to you around the clock, but in the difficult first weeks of your diet, when you feel that you might lapse back to old habits at any moment, you need help from someone who is dependable. The helper you choose should understand that your situation is unpredictable—you can't schedule a crisis of confidence. And this individual needs to be patient—someone who responds to your concerns with indifference or ridicule is of no value.

Questions to Ask Your Helper

You also need to be sure your helper does not have an independent agenda when it comes to weight control. Ask yourself:

1. Does my helper really want me to succeed?

   Yes _____   No _____

2. Does this person have a hidden reason to see me fail?

   Yes _____   No _____

3. If my helper is overweight, is it possible that this person could be threatened by my attempts at weight control?

   Yes _____   No _____

4. If my helper has always been thin, will he or she be able to empathize with my struggle?

   Yes _____   No _____

5. Is this person sensitive enough to know when to give me breathing space?

   Yes _____   No _____

You can feel most comfortable with the helper you have chosen if the answers to all five questions match these:

1. Yes
2. No
3. No
4. Yes
5. Yes

If one or more of the responses do not match, you should think about choosing another helper.

An Open Letter to My Helper

Drawing on the experiences of the people in my practice, as well as tools that have been developed by counselors who specialize in food problems, I've written an open letter for you to use as a guide. You may want to write something similar to the person you are asking to be your helper. (The comments in parentheses are addressed to you and are intended to help you clarify your requests.)

Dear Helper:

I have a problem with my weight and I'm committed to a new approach to dieting that will put me in control. I am writing to ask if you can help me.

Let's start by being honest. I am overweight. But there's nothing wrong with me and I need you to understand that. The messages in our culture suggest that people who are fat are not fully deserving members of society. That's an attitude we should work together to change. Genetic and metabolic factors in my life make it very hard for me to control my weight. Treat me the way you would treat anyone who is trying to overcome a chronic medical problem. *(You might want to tell your helper how to refer to your weight problem—Do you think of yourself as "fat?" "Overweight?" "Heavy?" Feel free to suggest the language you prefer.)*

I know that I have some real problems with…*(Here is where you can describe your own situation in detail. Do you tend to overeat at social or business gatherings? When you feel under stress? Be candid.)*

I need to make some adjustments to my daily activities, especially in terms of what I eat, how I prepare my meals, and how much exercise I get. I'd be delighted if you could help me make those adjustments. *(Do you want your helper to come to your house to cook with you?*

Or to participate in your new exercise routines? Be specific about your needs.)

I am going to try very hard to stick to my new routines, but you will probably see me lapse back to old patterns from time to time. Have patience with me—even when I don't have patience with myself. *(When you get a little careless, do you want a gentle reminder from your helper? Or do you prefer this person to stay silent?)*

I plan to be successful at this. If you want to give me an incentive to persevere or reward me for my success, please don't do it with food. *(You might want to suggest other ways you'd like to be encouraged. One idea is to set a goal and make a date to celebrate when you achieve it.)*

This is a long-range program. Please don't ever ask, "Are you still on that diet?" I'm making major, permanent changes in my life. I don't intend to go back to my old habits.

You mean a lot to me. Because I trust you, I'm asking for your help. If you're not able to help, I'll understand. But please be honest with me. I'm opening up a painful part of myself to you and I need your respect.

Thank you.

Being this open can be very difficult, especially if your weight has been an excuse to hide from the world. But if you learn to be candid with someone you care about, you may be able to get valuable support.

CHOOSING A WEIGHT CONTROL DOCTOR

Until relatively recently, very few physicians specialized in the area of weight control. Many who called themselves "diet doctors" operated at the fringes of the medical community. Fortunately, things are changing and there are now well-qualified and talented doctors available in many communities. Many are doctors of internal medicine, like myself; others specialize in endocrinology or gastroenterology.

Although this book provides all the information you need to lose weight, some people prefer to follow the Getting Healthy plan under the supervision of a doctor. If you think that will work best for you, I'm all for it. The safest way to find a qualified physician with expertise in weight control is to ask for a recommendation. Your own doctor or a friend with a weight problem (preferably someone who has gotten his or her own weight under control) may be good referral sources. If there is a hospital or medical school in your area, call to ask whether someone in the nutrition or endocrinology department can make a referral for you. Some institutions now have comprehensive weight control clinics with programs similar to the one that I have developed at New York Hospital/Cornell Medical Center.

After you have lined up some medical prospects, schedule a consultation to discuss possible treatment options. Any credible physician should be willing to talk to you, usually for a modest fee. Sometimes another person in the office will handle this discussion. If you feel awkward asking doctors certain questions, such as the extent of their experience, you may be able to discuss them with someone else in the office.

Don't be shy about asking for what you want—remember, you are the consumer shopping for the product. Be prepared to describe your own goals and be clear about what you are looking for in a physician. Because weight control is such a personal subject, you need to feel comfortable and open with your doctor. The ability to communicate in a climate of mutual respect is the key to building a successful working relationship.

Questions to Ask about the Weight Control Doctor

What is your weight control philosophy?

There are many different approaches to weight control, so make sure your doctor's attitude is in synch with your own. Some physicians custom-tailor their treatment to each patient. Others use a fairly uniform program with everyone. Find out if your doctor accepts my three-point Getting Healthy plan of diet, exercise, and behavioral changes. If not, ask why. My framework is flexible enough so that most physicians will be comfortable with it.

Do you work closely with other health professionals?

I believe it is difficult to build a successful weight control program without a comprehensive model. I strongly favor finding a physician who has well-established and ongoing relationships with a psychologist or some other professional counselor, an exercise specialist, and a nutritionist and who is willing to make referrals for you, as necessary.

Are you involved with weight control support groups?

Many physicians will refer you to mutual support groups where you can talk with other people in situations similar to yours. Even if a support group does not appeal to you right now, you may change your mind in the future and it is nice to know it is available.

Will you be providing my health care as well as helping me control my weight?

Find out if this physician focuses exclusively on weight loss or expects to manage any associated health-care problems as well. Make sure you are getting the kind of care you want.

What is your educational background? What was the last continuing education course that you took?

Some physicians claim to be experts in treating weight control problems but have had no training in the field. Make sure your doctor has some specific, and recent, educational credentials related to weight issues.

How long have you been involved in weight control?

There is no hard-and-fast rule here, but it is best to find a doctor who has had ample experience with problems like yours.

How many people do you see in one week?

You want someone with a steady practice, but not someone who is overextended. Make sure this individual will be able to devote enough time to meet your needs. Beware of diet "mills."

Do you treat people with severe eating disorders?

Some physicians have a lot of experience with disorders such as anorexia and bulimia; others prefer to make referrals. Find out whether you can get the care you need.

How long do you anticipate we will be working together?

Six months is the minimum time needed to address most weight problems. Beware of someone who promises you swifter results. On the other hand, achieving an initial weight-loss goal should not be an open-ended task. The best approach is to set a specific goal and then to renegotiate your commitment once that has been achieved.

How long do your patients maintain their weight loss?

Obviously, you want to find a doctor who has a good long-term success rate, but statistics may be hard to come by.

How frequently do you see your patients?

Some physicians schedule weekly appointments whereas others prefer biweekly or monthly appointments. Individual needs vary, depending on the complexity of your problem and the type of treatment you are receiving.

What is your fee?

The staff in the doctor's office should be able to give you a specific breakdown of costs and help you determine what will be covered by your health insurance plan.

What is your policy for canceled sessions?

Some physicians ask to be paid for any canceled session, either because they will not otherwise fill the appointment slot or because they believe such a policy encourages people to honor their commitments. Others have a cancelation policy that allows you to reschedule an appointment at no cost, as long as you provide twenty-four or forty-eight hours' notice. Still others try to be very flexible in order to accommodate the demands of a long-term relationship. Establish your physician's policy from the outset.

Will I need to purchase products from you?

Some offices may sell products at a modest markup because they are difficult to find. However, you should beware of professionals who insist that you buy anything from them. Unfortunately, the weight control field still has its share of unseemly practitioners who are more interested in selling you merchandise than in treating your weight problem. In most instances, medication you need as part of your treatment should be prescribed, rather than dispensed in the physician's office.

What to Expect from a Weight Control Doctor

Once you choose a doctor, you will schedule a first appointment to assess your overall health status and outline a weight-loss strategy. In my own practice, I begin by asking a lot of questions about medication use, stress levels, and medical history and I try to learn more about each individual's eating patterns.

The next step is to develop an individualized diet plan and an exercise program. Many medical professionals will be quite comfortable using the Getting Healthy meal plans in Part Four, or something quite similar. Any recommended meal plan should be based on sound nutritional principles and structured to achieve a weight loss of no more than 1 pound per week—or, 1 percent of your body weight per week at the most.

I insist that everyone in my practice return for regular follow-up appointments so that I can monitor their progress. And I believe a good physician never gives up. If the first effort to control your weight does not begin to show results after two months, a different approach may be appropriate. Your meal plans can be redesigned and you can alter or intensify your exercise regimen. If your weight problem is especially severe, your physician may even consider a liquid diet, drug therapy, or surgery—more radical alternatives that require ongoing medical supervision.

Warning: When to Change Doctors

No doctor should promise you a cure for your weight problem or offer any sort of weight-loss wonder drug. It would be wonderful if such things existed, but unfortunately, they don't—at least not yet. Think seriously about finding an alternate source of medical care if your doctor:

❖ Guarantees that you will lose a certain number of pounds within some time period

❖ Promises that you will be able to keep off lost weight effortlessly

❖ Prescribes combinations of diet pills, tranquilizers, and sleep aids

❖ Treats you with diuretics or thyroid pills

❖ Recommends megadoses of vitamins or a diet plan that doesn't meet your daily nutrient requirements

Any of these practices can be extremely harmful to your health.

WORKING WITH A REGISTERED DIETITIAN

If you are having trouble living within the limits of your diet, consulting a registered dietitian is another option to consider. Although most people are referred to a dietitian by their physician, it is perfectly appropriate to consult someone on your own. In private, one-on-one sessions, a dietitian will educate you about nutrition, examine your food choices, and help you design meal plans that are healthy and appropriate.

Contact the American Dietetic Association (ADA) (see Resources) for a referral to someone in your community. Members of the American Dietetic Association are highly qualified and current on the latest nutritional thinking because they are required to take 75 educational credits every five years. If you have a particular type of eating disorder—binging or anorexia, for example—you may want to ask the ADA about specialists or find a very focused program.

It is just as important to feel comfortable with your dietitian as with your doctor. Once again, you will be discussing your eating habits in intimate detail and will want to work with someone who does not make you feel embarrassed. It is completely appropriate to ask about the dietitian's philosophy and approach.

Most dietitians will schedule an initial session with you to discuss your background and your needs. You may be encouraged to keep a food diary and to bring it with you to every session. (If you've already started the Getting Healthy plan, you know all about this; see Chapter 7.) At first, you will probably meet weekly, or every other week. Once you have a program in place that seems to be working, you can cut back your visits to about once a month.

A session with a dietitian usually runs thirty to forty minutes. Typical costs are $100 to $150 for the first visit and $50 to $75 after that. This can become a substantial investment, but many health insurance policies cover at least some of the fee, particularly if your weight problem puts you at high risk for medical complications.

THE VALUE OF A COUNSELOR

Because I believe the psychological dimensions of weight control are so important, counseling services are an essential component of the comprehensive care provided at my clinic. A detached and knowledgeable outsider may be able to help you confront deep-seated, and possibly long-buried, personal problems that often interfere with weight loss. The process can be painful, but for many people it is essential.

Understanding Your Choices

It is up to you to decide whether you prefer to consult a psychiatrist, psychologist, social worker, or some other qualified counselor:

- ❖ A psychiatrist is a physician who can prescribe medication. This may be appropriate for some people who are extremely depressed or anxious, but it is not necessary for everyone.

- ❖ Psychologists are either licensed or certified on a state-by-state basis. Psychologists have substantial scientific training and are required in most, but not all, states to have doctoral degrees.

- ❖ Clinical social workers, sometimes referred to as psychiatric social workers, are usually licensed or certified by some sort of statewide credentialing process. Generally, they are required to have master's degrees.

- ❖ Mental health counselors have a wide variety of qualifications. In general, their training tends to be a little less stringent and formal than that of the other health professionals described here, but many counselors are well qualified to give you the support you need. Some states require mental health counselors to be licensed.

Regardless of who you consult, your goal is the same: to stop the destructive behaviors that prevent you from gaining control of your weight.

Therapeutic Styles

There are a number of different therapeutic techniques that are effective for weight control and it is important to find one that feels comfortable to you. Many counselors use an eclectic mix of styles, with psychodynamic and behavioral techniques among the most popular:

- ❖ The **psychodynamic approach** relies primarily on an intensive dialogue between client and counselor. The theory is that by identifying and talking about incidents from your past, often going all the way back to childhood, you will gain sufficient insight to break old patterns.

- ❖ The **behavioral approach** focuses exclusively on changing troubling behavior, rather than understanding its origins. A behaviorist will teach you concrete ways to cope with anxiety and other counterproductive emotions, and will help you alter your automatic responses, such as overeating when you feel depressed.

Questions to Ask the Counselor

Once you have identified several candidates, schedule a consultation with at least two or three people. Regardless of the counselor's academic credentials, you have to feel comfortable in order to be able to share confidences. Any qualified professional understands this and will willingly give you an initial consultation, usually for a modest fee. Here are some questions you should ask:

Do you have experience or training in dealing with weight problems or eating disorders?

Have you dealt with problems that are similar to mine?

What is your treatment style?

How do you feel about group therapy? What do you consider to be its pros and its cons for me?

How long do you think my treatment will last? How do you decide when to provide short-term guidance and when long-term therapy is more appropriate? (Short-term therapy has been gaining popularity for weight control problems and works well for many people.)

After the Consultation

It is not necessary for you and your counselor to agree on everything, but you should leave the introductory session feeling confident and comfortable with this person. Once your meeting is finished, ask yourself:

Did the counselor seem to understand the nature of my problems?

Did this person really listen?

Did this person ask appropriate and pointed questions?

(Remember, if your counselor asks questions that seem unrelated to weight control, it may be because the counselor sees connections that you have not considered.)

Most counselors want to meet with their clients on a weekly basis, and fees vary greatly, depending on credentials and the region of the country in which you are located. Many health insurance plans will cover the cost of some mental health services.

COMMERCIAL WEIGHT CONTROL PROGRAMS

Unfortunately, most commercial weight control programs are not especially helpful. They aren't generally run by licensed professionals and they are more concerned with quick weight loss than with weight maintenance. Beware of "white coat" syndrome—in a thinly disguised bit of chicanery, some weight control programs insist their staff wear clothing that resembles that of medical personnel. Also, most commercial programs tend to emphasize the product they are selling, and that means most people won't learn how to avoid regaining weight over the long term.

Most objective evaluations of commercial weight programs have reached the same conclusion. The American Board of Nutrition says: "With rare exceptions, none of the popular commercially available programs for treating obesity are based on current scientific knowledge. They could no longer promise rapid weight loss if they were."

Consumer Reports seconded that opinion in its June 1993 issue in which it rated numerous commercial approaches: "There is no evidence that commercial weight-loss programs help most people achieve significant, permanent weight loss. If you want or need to lose weight, you would probably do well to try and reduce on your own, or through a free hospital-based program, before spending money on a commercial weight-loss center."

Weight Watchers was one important exception to this generally negative report. According to *Consumer Reports*, 74 percent of the people who tried a Weight Watchers program were satisfied with their weight loss and more than half of them remained satisfied six months later. Many people I work with speak highly of Weight Watchers, which is particularly good at providing information about meal planning and food exchanges.

Questions to Ask About Commercial Programs

If you are interested in learning more about any commercial weight-loss program in your area, be sure to ask some of these questions before putting down your hard-earned cash:

Does this program make scientific and common sense?

Does it suit my special psychological, social, and physiological needs?

How much education about nutrition and physiology is included?

What is the recommended rate of weight loss?

Is the diet nutritionally balanced? How flexible are the food choices?

Does the program encourage a reasonable level of exercise?

Are sources of group motivation, or individual, one-on-one support available?

Is the program medically supervised? Will my progress be monitored by a physician?

Does the program offer access to any professionals, including dietitians and counselors?

Does the staff have any specialized training in weight control?

What percentage of people complete the program once they begin?

Is there a maintenance plan once I reach my target weight?

How many people maintain their weight after one year? After five years?

How much will this cost? Do I have to buy any special foods, devices, or books? (You may find that the cost of a medical professional is no higher than a commercial program.)

How does the program advertise itself? Would your own doctor recommend it?

PART THREE

THE NUTS AND BOLTS OF DIETING

6

LEARNING GOOD
FOOD HABITS

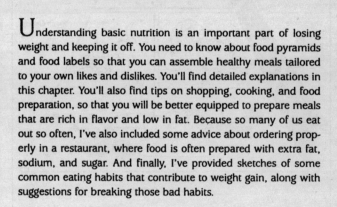

Understanding basic nutrition is an important part of losing weight and keeping it off. You need to know about food pyramids and food labels so that you can assemble healthy meals tailored to your own likes and dislikes. You'll find detailed explanations in this chapter. You'll also find tips on shopping, cooking, and food preparation, so that you will be better equipped to prepare meals that are rich in flavor and low in fat. Because so many of us eat out so often, I've also included some advice about ordering properly in a restaurant, where food is often prepared with extra fat, sodium, and sugar. And finally, I've provided sketches of some common eating habits that contribute to weight gain, along with suggestions for breaking those bad habits.

THE FOOD PYRAMID

Two food pyramids provide important dietary guidance to consumers. One was developed by the U.S. Department of Agriculture. The other, known as the Mediterranean diet, was a collaboration of the Center for Nutrition at the Harvard School of

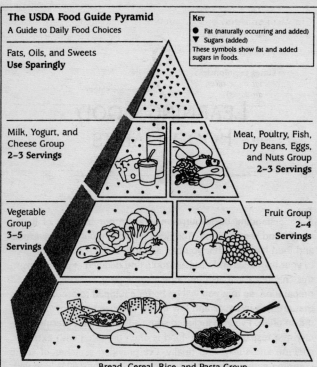

The USDA Food Guide Pyramid
A Guide to Daily Food Choices

KEY
● Fat (naturally occurring and added)
▼ Sugars (added)
These symbols show fat and added sugars in foods.

Fats, Oils, and Sweets
Use Sparingly

Milk, Yogurt, and Cheese Group
2–3 Servings

Meat, Poultry, Fish, Dry Beans, Eggs, and Nuts Group
2–3 Servings

Vegetable Group
3–5 Servings

Fruit Group
2–4 Servings

Bread, Cereal, Rice, and Pasta Group
6–11 Servings

What is the Food Guide Pyramid?
The Pyramid is an outline of what to eat each day. It's not a rigid prescription, but a general guide that lets you choose a healthful diet that's right for you. The Pyramid calls for eating a variety of foods to get the nutrients you need and at the same time the right amount of calories to maintain a healthy weight. The Pyramid restricts fat, an important reminder to many Americans whose diets are too high in fat, especially saturated fat.

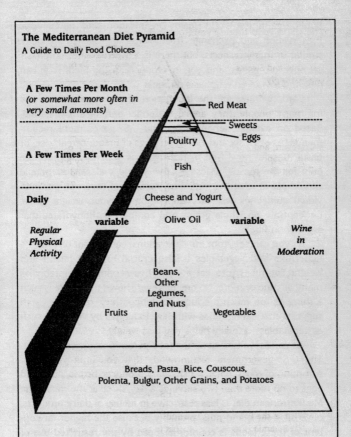

The Mediterranean Diet Pyramid
A Guide to Daily Food Choices

A Few Times Per Month
(or somewhat more often in very small amounts) — Red Meat

Sweets
Eggs
Poultry
Fish

A Few Times Per Week

Daily

Cheese and Yogurt

Regular Physical Activity   **variable**   Olive Oil   **variable**   *Wine in Moderation*

Beans, Other Legumes, and Nuts

Fruits   Vegetables

Breads, Pasta, Rice, Couscous, Polenta, Bulgur, Other Grains, and Potatoes

Source: Collaboration of the Center for Nutrition at the Harvard School of Public Health, World Health Organization, and Oldways Preservation & Exchange Trust.

Public Health, the World Health Organization, and the Oldways Preservation and Exchange Trust. These approaches are quite similar in many respects, but there is a much greater emphasis on olive oil, grains, and yogurt products in the Mediterranean diet and less of an emphasis on meat.

Carbohydrates are the foundation of both approaches, and for many people, they are an essential part of smart eating. Based on average serving sizes, the U.S. government recommends between six and eleven servings of bread, cereal, rice, or pasta. Careful now! The higher figure is generally appropriate only for the most physically active young males. Most people should eat at least the minimum number of servings, but individual guidelines will vary depending on your weight goals. Concentrate on whole grains and complex carbohydrates that are high in fiber.

As you can see from the illustrations, eating a lot of vitamin-rich fruits and vegetables is also crucial to good health and weight control. Try to eat at least five servings, preferably as many as nine or more. No one has ever shown that there is such a thing as too much produce. To the contrary, recent research suggests that eating foods with fewer calories by volume—such as vegetables—actually helps you lose weight.

As you move further up the food pyramid, exercise restraint. The U.S. government recommends that you limit your consumption of meat, poultry, fish, dairy products, beans, nuts, and eggs to no more than two servings a day, three at the most. The Mediterranean diet is less restrictive in its use of dairy products, olive oil, beans, and nuts, probably because the higher fat content of these foods is counterbalanced by the restricted use of most animal products—in this pyramid, consumption of fish and poultry is limited to a few times per week and red meats are not eaten more than a few times a month.

Both approaches reflect the need to restrict protein consumption to modest levels, which is relatively new advice. Historically, people have been worried about eating *enough* protein, which is probably why Americans developed such a passion for meat. Up to a point, this was an appropriate concern because the storehouse of protein in your body is vulnerable, and if you do not consume enough protein, muscle loss can result. Today, however, excess protein is a much more relevant issue for most Americans, especially since many high-protein foods are also high in fat.

Menu Plan I of the Getting Healthy program, the low-fat, high-carbohydrate approach, fits within the framework of both food pyramids. Menu Plan II, the lower glycemic index approach, strays slightly from the pyramid recommendations because it reduces simple carbohydrates and starches. That's a complicating factor, but it just illustrates one of my cardinal beliefs about healthy eating and weight control: No single approach works for everyone. In the rapidly evolving field of nutrition, I wouldn't be surprised if some of my recommendations are modified in the years to come. The food pyramids are just guides, so don't let them win over common sense or your own experiences.

THE NEW FOOD LABEL

Beginning in the spring of 1994, the Food and Drug Administration required all food manufacturers to use a standard Nutrition Facts label on their products. The new label is a terrific source of information about what you are eating. Here is what it tells you:

- ❖ How much fat, cholesterol, sodium, sugar, fiber, protein, and other nutrients are in a serving of food
- ❖ How much of the day's recommended intake of certain nutrients, such as vitamins, calcium, and iron, you are consuming in a serving of food
- ❖ How each food fits into an overall healthy diet
- ❖ Information to compare the nutritional value of similar products

And there's more good news. Label descriptions like "low-calorie," "fat-free," "lite," and "lean" finally have specific, legally

THE NEW FOOD LABEL AT A GLANCE

The new food label will carry an up-to-date, easier-to-use nutrition information guide. The guide will serve as a key to help in planning a healthy diet.*

Serving sizes are now more consistent across product lines, stated in both household and metric measures, and reflect the amounts people actually eat.

The list of nutrients covers those most important to the health of today's consumers, most of whom need to worry about getting *too much* of certain items (fat, for example), rather than too few vitamins, as in the past.

The label of larger packages may tell the number of calories per gram of fat, carbohydrate, and protein.

Nutrition Facts

Serving Size ½ cup (114g)
Servings Per Container 4

Amount Per Serving

Calories 90   Calories from Fat 30

% Daily Value*

Total Fat 3g	5%
Saturated Fat 0g	0%
Cholesterol 0mg	0%
Sodium 300mg	13%
Total Carbohydrate 13g	4%
Dietary Fiber 3g	12%
Sugars 3g	
Protein 3g	

Vitamin A 80%	•	Vitamin C 60%	
Calcium 4%	•	Iron 4%	

* Percent Daily Values are based on a 2,000 calorie diet. Your daily values may be higher or lower depending on your calorie needs:

	Calories:	2,000	2,500
Total Fat	Less than	65g	80g
Sat Fat	Less than	20g	25g
Cholesterol	Less than	300mg	300mg
Sodium	Less than	2,400mg	2,400mg
Total Carbohydrate		300g	375g
Dietary Fiber		25g	30g

Calories per gram:
Fat 9 • Carbohydrate 4 • Protein 4

New title signals that the label contains the newly required information.

Calories from fat are now shown on the label to help consumers meet dietary guidelines that recommend people get no more than 30 percent of their calories from fat each day.

% Daily Value shows how a food fits into the overall daily diet. It puts all nutrients on the same scale, so consumers trying to eat a more healthful diet will no longer have to remember what number is low for fat, saturated fat, cholesterol, and sodium, but can simply look for 5 or less on an individual food.

Daily Values are also something new. Some are maximums, as with fat (less than 65 grams); others are minimums, as with carbohydrate (300 grams *or more*). The daily values for a 2,000- and 2,500-calorie diet must be listed on the label of larger packages. Individuals should adjust the values to fit their own calorie intake.

*This label is only a sample. Exact specifications are in the final rules.
Source: Food and Drug Administration, 1994.

defined meanings. Manufacturers can no longer claim a product is a "good source" of a desirable nutrient unless it really has a significant percentage of the total day's requirement. And a food that is labeled "healthy" has to be low in fat, saturated fat, sodium, and cholesterol (see "What the Labeling Claims Mean" on page 89).

I'm very excited about the new food labels. They provide a crucial service to the American consumer. If you read them and base your shopping decisions on what they say, you'll be making a major contribution to your own weight control efforts. Don't be misled, however. Just because a food is labeled "nonfat" does not mean it has fewer calories than the original version. Read *all* the information on the label.

TIPS FOR REDUCING DIETARY FAT

Many researchers are convinced that the average American diet contains too much fat for good health. Moreover, fat is much higher in calories by weight than other nutrients. Consider this:

- ❖ 1 gram of fat = 9 calories
- ❖ 1 gram of carbohydrates = 4 calories
- ❖ 1 gram of protein = 4 calories

What does that mean to you? It means you can eat a much higher volume of food if it is low in fat. You can put a tablespoon of butter on your bread or you can eat 3 ounces of shrimp. You can have a cup of cooked pasta or seven deep-fried tortilla chips. The calorie counts are the same. When you eat a low-fat diet, you can actually eat more in volume and weigh less. And there is a huge fringe benefit—you greatly reduce your risk of coronary artery disease and other medical problems associated with fatty foods.

The food label tells you how many grams of fat are contained in an average serving and what percentage of total calories are derived from fat. These are the Golden Rules of fat consumption:

- ❖ Fewer than 30 percent of a day's calories should come from fat. Many physicians believe that less than 25 percent is wiser.

❖ Fewer than 10 percent of your calories should come from
   saturated fat. (Saturated fats are contained in meat and
   dairy products and certain plant oils, such as coconut oil
   and palm oil.)

Many processed foods grossly exceed these limits. Buttered
popcorn, for example, derives two-thirds of its calories from fat.
And fat is the source of 70 percent of the calories in some commercially packaged cookies.

If you are scrupulous about reducing the fat in your diet, you
will quickly see the results in your waistline. Fortunately, you can
now buy many reduced-fat and no-fat products—such as sour
cream, cottage cheese, and even ice cream, to name a few—and
slash your fat grams and calorie count at the same time.

By the way, I'm not suggesting you eliminate fat altogether.
A little fat may help you control your weight because it satisfies
the body's fat-craving mechanism and slows down the digestive
process, leaving you feeling fuller and more satisfied. Some people actually feel anxious if they do not eat enough fat. But very
few of us have to worry about that problem. The challenge is
much more likely to be reducing fat intake.

Remember that the total number of calories you consume still
counts. Many people have taken the messages about a low-fat diet
to heart, yet keep on gaining weight. Why? Because they are eating too much. Pasta is great, but if you polish off a pound of it in
one sitting, you are going to keep getting heavier, even if that
sauce has no fat at all. Likewise, you can't get thin eating an entire
box of cookies, even if it doesn't contain a single gram of fat.

TIPS FOR SHOPPING

Danger lurks when you walk into a supermarket. The aisles are
laden with heavily processed food and tempting instant meals
filled with sodium and fat. It takes a combination of knowledge
and discipline to buy wisely. Here are some tips:

❖ **Shop the walls.** Most supermarkets deliberately organize
   their merchandise so that you are tempted to buy the con-

venience foods that provide most of their profit. The savvy supermarket shopper "shops the walls," walking around the edge of the store to find fresh food, including bread, produce, dairy products, meats, poultry, and fish.

❖ **Know what you have come for.** Don't walk into a supermarket until you have planned your menus and made a shopping list. Then, stick to it.

❖ **Always shop on a full stomach.** If you are not hungry, you are less likely to give in to cravings when you shop.

❖ **Buy prepared foods cautiously.** Ideally, I'd like you to cook your meals from scratch, so that you have more control over the ingredients. I understand this isn't possible, but it is important to find out exactly what is in any prepared food you buy.

❖ **Experiment with new products.** The new food label, combined with growing consumer concerns about eating right, has led to an explosion of tasty new foods in the supermarket. They may help put some variety in your diet.

❖ **Read food labels carefully.** Be especially careful about buying foods that are labeled low-fat—often the manufacturer adds extra sodium or sugar to retain flavor. And don't make any assumptions—for example, some brands of turkey hot dogs, which you might think would be healthier than beef hot dogs, actually contain more fat.

❖ **Dispose of unhealthy foods.** Getting the right food into your house is only half the battle; getting the wrong food out is the other half. Clean out your cabinets before starting the Getting Healthy plan and throw away any foods that are high in fat or sugar.

TIPS FOR COOKING

Prepare your kitchen for low-fat cooking and eating with these suggestions:

❖ **Purchase an accurate scale with ounce measurements.** A scale will help you control portion sizes. Newer designs are more stable than traditional scales and they hold odd-shaped containers without toppling over.

❖ **Make sure your knives are sharpened.** There's nothing more frustrating than trying to cut the right portion size with a dull knife. And it is more satisfying to eat a lot of thinly sliced foods than to gobble down food in large chunks.

❖ **Grill or broil meats and vegetables.** Buying a grill or hibachi for the backyard or apartment terrace can help you prepare healthy, tasty meats and vegetables. You can also use an electric or stove-top indoor grill or the oven broiler—these don't duplicate the flavor of foods cooked outside, but it is much better than frying. (When you are grilling, be careful not to char or burn your food, which may be carcinogenic.)

❖ **Use skewers.** Vegetable, fish, and meat skewers are fast to prepare, allow you to control fat content and portion size, and make food look very appetizing.

❖ **Prepare only as much food as you are going to eat.** If a recipe feeds six to eight people, and you are cooking for four, reduce the recipe by at least one-third. Otherwise, the extra portions may get eaten.

❖ **Cook with nonstick skillets or nonstick cooking sprays.** Products such as Pam, and butter substitutes such as Butter Buds, are much lower in calories and fat than butter and oil. If you need cooking fat, use only canola or olive oil, which are monounsaturated fats and appear to lower the risk of coronary disease. (Olive oil imparts a hearty flavor to foods, so it won't be appropriate for all your recipes.)

❖ **Weigh meats after cooking.** Three ounces of cooked meat is equal to 4 ounces of raw meat. Three ounces of cooked meat is about the size of a deck of cards.

❖ **Prepare snacks in advance.** When you are hungry, you are likely to reach for anything that is fast and convenient. Be prepared with ready-to-eat foods—such as low-fat crackers, air-popped popcorn, pretzels, or cut-up vegetables—stored in small-portion bags at home and work.

TIPS FOR EATING AT HOME

When you decide to get serious about weight control, you may have to learn a whole new way of eating. Here are some guidelines:

❖ **Eat slowly.** Put down your fork between bites. Pause as you eat.

❖ **Don't do anything else while you are eating.** Concentrate on the food on your table and learn to enjoy every morsel.

❖ **Eat in the same place every day.** At home, eat in the dining room or kitchen, not in front of the television or in bed. At work, eat in a lunchroom, or at a table, not at your desk. That will help you concentrate on what you are doing.

❖ **Eat breakfast.** Some people complain that eating the full breakfast I recommend makes them ravenous later in the day. If you are not accustomed to a full meal in the morning, this may occur at first, but the feeling seldom lasts long, and once you adjust you will find that a healthy breakfast probably helps you eat less. You may want to eat your first meal a little later in the morning and delay lunch until midafternoon.

❖ **Don't skip meals or snacks.** By spreading out your caloric intake over the day, you'll fend off food cravings, keep your metabolic rate and blood sugar up, and avoid the crankiness and fatigue often associated with dieting.

❖ **Drink liquids.** If you drink a glass of seltzer or ice water before your meal and sip on another glass as you eat, you will feel more full and may be less tempted to overeat.

❖ **Stock up on low-calorie drinks.** Sometimes, people think they are hungry when the real problem is thirst. Just the act of pouring a drink for yourself may consume some of the nervous energy that is often part of overeating. Keep a nice assortment of flavored seltzer and diet beverages in your refrigerator.

❖ **Avoid trigger foods.** Some people find it almost impossible not to consume excess amounts of certain fried, salty, or sweet foods, such as ice cream, corn chips, chocolate, and candy. Generally, the best way to avoid overeating these trigger foods is not to eat them at all. For now, the advertising line, "Bet you can't eat just one," is all too true.

❖ **Ask someone to clean up.** If you can, try to arrange for someone else to clear the table and wash the dishes, especially during the first few weeks of your diet. That may help you avoid the temptation of leftovers.

❖ **Satisfy your sweet tooth.** Fresh fruits and low-fat desserts may ease sugar cravings. Just be sure to watch calories and fat content. Again, the food label is your best guide to this information. You may also want to check out some of the dessert suggestions in Part Four. But know thyself—if you can't eat just a little, it is wisest to eat none at all.

TIPS FOR EATING IN RESTAURANTS

Because eating out is usually a treat, it easily becomes an excuse to indulge. "Just this once," you say before succumbing to temptation. Unfortunately, restaurant meals pose special problems for weight control because they are typically 40 percent higher in calories and fat than the same meals cooked at home. It is possible to eat sensibly at restaurants, but only if you plan carefully and are very disciplined. Here are some tips:

❖ **Plan your meal in advance.** It is much easier to think about what you're going to order before you get into the restaurant than to make wise choices once the menu arrives.

❖ **Focus on the conversation.** Concentrate on your dinner companions rather than all the food that is available to you.

❖ **Be assertive.** Don't be afraid to ask how food is prepared or how big the portions are.

❖ **Send food back to the kitchen.** If the waiter tells you a dish is low in fat but it arrives soaked in butter or oil, don't hesitate to complain.

❖ **Make special requests.** Most foods can be just as tasty with much less fat. Ask if the chef is willing to prepare your meal with half the butter, oil, or fat that is normally used.

❖ **Request that dressings, gravy, and sauces be served on the side.** This will give you control over how much you use.

❖ **Limit your drinking.** Alcohol adds calories to your meal, weakens your willpower, and may even impede your body's ability to burn fat.

❖ **Watch the extras.** A cheese topping, sour cream with your baked potato, or a side order of onion rings can send fat consumption and calorie counts into the stratosphere.

❖ **You don't have to eat everything on your plate.** Regardless of what your mother may have told you, no one benefits if you insist on finishing all of the food on your plate. Stop when you feel full.

BREAKING BAD HABITS

Some people overeat because they are having a great time at a party. Others tend to overeat because they weren't invited. Perhaps your lifestyle is filled with business meals, social engagements, and family gatherings, and food is an important part of the activity. Or you may be eating for the complex psychological reasons we have discussed earlier, typically using food to fill a feeling of emptiness, rather than to satisfy physical hunger or a nutritional need.

If you recognize your own eating patterns in the descriptions below, don't be discouraged. I've also included some useful tips that will help you break bad habits once you identify them.

Bingers and Grazers

Bingers typically eat big meals very quickly whereas grazers tend to consume small amounts of food throughout the day. If you fit either one of these profiles, chances are you are having trouble shaking a powerful urge to finish everything in sight. Any package of food within your reach is fair game—and once opened, it is likely that every morsel in the package will be consumed.

If you binge . . .

Control the amount of food you prepare. For some people, the best approach is to keep very little food in the house. Of course, that means making more trips to the store, so this technique only works if you are a careful shopper. Another good trick is to munch on healthy food as you prepare a meal—some cut-up vegetables with a low-fat dip often satisfy the common urge to nibble while cooking.

I also tell binge eaters to prepare small portions and to seal away extra food before sitting down to eat the meal. Every calorie safely put away in your refrigerator or cupboard is one less calorie that you won't store as body fat.

Nighttime Eaters

Perhaps you eat very little during the day and then consume huge quantities of food at night. There are many reasons why. In some cases, you may simply be too busy during the day to squeeze in a meal. Or you may be fooling yourself into thinking you can lose weight by starving yourself all day—only to find that at night, you are ravenous. By then, you rarely have the patience to prepare a healthy meal, so you are likely to gobble up anything that is quick and easy, regardless of the fat and nutrient content.

Nighttime eaters face three problems. First, unplanned meals aren't likely to be very healthy. Second, packing in a lot of food at night could pose a challenge to the body's ability to burn calories, although this has not been scientifically proven. Third, and perhaps most importantly, your chance to compensate for the excess calories is gone—if you overeat at lunch, you can eat less at dinner, but if you eat too much too late, your whole day's calorie count may be shot.

If you eat mostly at night . . .
Try to change your eating patterns so that you have at least one substantial meal during the day. Another effective trick is to prepare foods ahead of time, so that when you arrive home hungry, there are healthy snacks or complete dinners that you can reheat quickly.

Big-Meal Eaters

Does your work or social life center around food? This is a common problem these days. You may attend a lot of lunch and dinner business meetings or travel frequently, where high-fat restaurant meals are a regular part of your life. Or you may attend frequent family gatherings, which often present opportunities to overindulge. While your metabolism can cope with occasional excess consumption, your weight set point will begin to creep up if the big-meal pattern never changes.

If you eat big meals in business and social settings . . .
The best way to cut back on big meals is to plan ahead. Keep in mind that you walk into temptation every time you walk into a restaurant. Steer yourself to avoid tempting, but fatty, appetizers and entrees. Think positive thoughts about the low-fat substitutes that give you both eating pleasure and the satisfaction of sticking to the Getting Healthy program.

It is perfectly appropriate to ask for help and support from business associates and family. Tell them that you are working hard to control your weight and suggest getting together in settings where food is not the main focus of attention. Most people will be glad to oblige.

Comfort Eaters

On one occasion or another, almost all of us eat to comfort ourselves, not because we are hungry. Feelings of anxiety, depression, and loneliness are especially likely to lead to overeating.
Unfortunately, the foods that make you feel better often contain
high amounts of fat and sugar. At moments of stress, you may
find it almost impossible to resist the temptation of eating those
foods.

If you are a comfort eater . . .
You may be able to satisfy your cravings for comfort foods in
small doses. Some people can only stay away from comfort
foods by adopting an all-or-nothing approach, but if you are luck-
ier, you may be able to eat a small amount of a special treat and
feel content. Stick with foods that you can consume in quantities
of less than 100 calories and you won't have to deal with any
guilt afterward.

Drinkers

Alcohol presents several problems to people who are trying to
control their weight. First, it has almost no nutritional value—an
alcoholic beverage is almost entirely empty calories. Second, scientists are exploring the theory that alcohol suppresses your
body's ability to burn fat. If that theory is right, you may wind
up storing more calories as fat if you drink with meals.

    Alcohol also has the tendency to lessen your willpower. And
you can't control your weight effectively if you've lost the
strength to say no. Drinking is probably the single most common cause of hard-to-overcome lapses in weight control. And
many people who have successfully managed to maintain lost
weight find the pounds creeping back on when they drink.

If you are a drinker . . .
Take it easy on the alcohol consumption. My clients seem to do
better having a glass of wine *with* dinner rather than before it,
perhaps because they are better able to maintain willpower.
More than one drink a day is likely to get you into trouble.

WHAT THE LABELING CLAIMS MEAN

Sugar

Sugar-free: less than 0.5 grams per serving

Reduced sugar: at least 25 percent less sugar per serving than the usual product

Calories

Calorie-free: fewer than 5 calories per serving

Low calorie: 40 calories or less per serving

Reduced or fewer calories: at least 25 percent fewer calories per serving than the usual product

Fat

Fat-free: less than 0.5 grams of fat per serving

Saturated fat-free: less than 0.5 grams per serving

Low fat: 3 grams or less per serving

Low saturated fat: 1 gram or less per serving and not more than 15 percent of calories derived from saturated fatty acids

Reduced or less fat: at least 25 percent less fat per serving than the usual product

Cholesterol

Cholesterol-free: less than 2 milligrams of cholesterol and 2 grams or less of saturated fat per serving

Low cholesterol: 20 milligrams or less of cholesterol and 2 grams or less of saturated fat per serving

Reduced or less cholesterol: at least 25 percent less cholesterol per serving and 2 grams or less of saturated fat per serving than the usual product

Sodium

Sodium-free: less than 5 milligrams of sodium per serving

Low sodium: 140 milligrams or less per serving

Very low sodium: 35 milligrams or less per serving

Reduced or less sodium: at least 25 percent less sodium per serving than the usual product

Fiber

High fiber: 5 grams or more of fiber per serving

Good source of fiber: 2.5 grams to 4.9 grams per serving

More or added fiber: at least 2.5 grams per serving more than the usual product

Light or Lite

The label will clarify how this term is being used. The possibilities are:

Contains one-third fewer calories than the usual product

Contains one-half the fat of the usual product

Contains one-half the sodium of the usual product

Lean

Lean meats have less than 10 grams of fat, including less than 4 grams of saturated fat per serving.

Extra-lean meats have less than 5 grams of fat, including less than 2 grams of saturated fat per serving.

High

Foods that are "high" in a certain nutrient must contain 20 percent or more of the daily value of that nutrient.

Healthy

Healthy foods must be low in fat and saturated fat and a serving cannot contain more than 480 milligrams of sodium or more than 60 milligrams of cholesterol.

7

KEEPING A WEIGHT
CONTROL JOURNAL

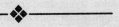

Now that you have some knowledge of nutrition and healthy
eating habits, you are ready to start monitoring your progress. A
Weight Control Journal is the cornerstone of success. The journal
is a comprehensive record of your measurements, weight goals,
food habits, and exercise routines. If you use the journal every
day, all through the day, you'll be able to identify the hidden
traps in your daily routine, see how you are responding to stress,
discover foods that trigger overeating, and learn how exercise
affects your appetite. You'll also be able to track your progress
over time and learn more about your deep-seated attitudes
toward body image and weight control.

I urge you to begin keeping a journal as soon as you commit
to the Getting Healthy program. Buy a small loose-leaf notebook
that allows you to add pages or move them around. Since you'll
be carrying the notebook with you everywhere, it is best to get
something small enough to fit into a handbag or knapsack—4
inches by 6 inches is a convenient and popular size. Be sure to
date all of your entries so that you can look back and make com-
parisons—for example, you might want to compare your food

diary with your exercise log in a week where you had trouble with your willpower.

The Weight Control Journal has five parts:

I.   Basic Measurements

II. Personal Weight History

III. The Food Diary

IV. The Exercise Log

V. Special Moments

It is not always easy to maintain this journal. You may hear an inner voice trying to discourage you from making new entries. Recognize that voice for what it is: a subconscious message to keep your weight up. This resistance is indirectly linked to the survival instincts that encourage us to store fat and make weight loss such a challenge.

Inevitably, the inner voice grows louder when you have strayed from your meal plans or stopped exercising regularly. Although this is the time when you are most likely to avoid telling the truth to your journal, it is also when it is most important to do so. By admitting your lapses and trying to explain them in writing, you are less likely to beat yourself up for being careless. You may even discover that, averaged over a week, you did not stray as far from your calorie or exercise goals as you thought.

I. BASIC MEASUREMENTS

The first section of your Weight Control Journal allows you to record baseline information about your height, weight, and other body measurements. For many years, the concept of an "ideal" body was reinforced by height and weight tables created by the Metropolitan Life Insurance Company. These widely reproduced tables set weight standards for people categorized as "small," "medium," and "large." Fortunately, these tables are no longer widely used to determine goal weights. They did a disservice to many of us by creating the impression that if your weight did not fall within a fairly narrow range, there was something abnormal about you. If you've still got those tables, toss them away and learn how to use the more useful tools described here instead.

First, enter your height and present weight in your journal.

Next, record your blood pressure and cholesterol count, including the level of high-density lipoproteins and triglycerides, each time you see a physician. These measurements provide a snapshot of your risk for medical problems, now and in the future.

Finally, measure and record your waist-to-hip ratio and body mass index (BMI).

Waist-to-Hip Ratio

As we discussed in Chapter 3, the waist-to-hip ratio helps you determine whether you are an "apple," which puts you at a higher risk for weight-related health problems, or a "pear," which is less medically risky, but the weight is harder to lose.

To calculate your waist-to-hip ratio, measure your waist 1 inch above the belly button and your hips at their widest diameter. Divide the hip measurement into the waist measurement. Say, for example, your waist size is 30 inches and your hips are 38 inches. Divide 30 by 38 and you get a waist-to-hip ratio of 0.79. That's a low-risk ratio—ideally, women have a ratio under 0.8 and men have a ratio below 0.95; the lower, the better.

Body Mass Index (BMI)

The Body Mass Index is a way to measure your weight, taking your height into account. Find your height and weight on the outer edges of the Body Mass Index Chart on pages 94–95. Now, follow the lines until you find the place where those measurements converge. That is your BMI.

Body Mass Index Chart

Weight		Height feet	4'10"	4'11"	5'	5'1"	5'2"	5'3"	5'4"	5'5"	5'6"	5'7"
		inches	58	59	60	61	62	63	64	65	66	67
		cm	147	150	152	155	157	160	163	165	168	170
lb	kg											
100	45.45		20.9	20.2	19.6	18.9	18.3	17.8	17.2	16.7	16.2	15.7
105	47.73		22.0	21.3	20.5	19.9	19.2	18.6	18.1	17.5	17.0	16.5
110	50.00		23.0	22.3	21.5	20.8	20.2	19.5	18.9	18.3	17.8	17.3
115	52.27		24.1	23.3	22.5	21.8	21.1	20.4	19.8	19.2	18.6	18.0
120	54.55		25.1	24.3	23.5	22.7	22.0	21.3	20.6	20.0	19.4	18.8
125	56.82		26.2	25.3	24.5	23.7	22.9	22.2	21.5	20.8	20.2	19.6
130	59.09		27.2	26.3	25.4	24.6	23.8	23.1	22.4	21.7	21.0	20.4
135	61.36		28.3	27.3	26.4	25.6	24.7	24.0	23.2	22.5	21.8	21.2
140	63.64		29.3	28.3	27.4	26.5	25.7	24.9	24.1	23.3	22.6	22.0
145	65.91		30.4	29.3	28.4	27.5	26.6	25.7	24.9	24.2	23.5	22.8
150	68.18		31.4	30.4	29.4	28.4	27.5	26.6	25.8	25.0	24.3	23.5
155	70.45		32.5	31.4	30.3	29.3	28.4	27.5	26.7	25.8	25.1	24.3
160	72.73		33.5	32.4	31.3	30.3	29.3	28.4	27.5	26.7	25.9	25.1
165	75.00		34.6	33.4	32.3	31.2	30.2	29.3	28.4	27.5	26.7	25.9
170	77.27		35.6	34.4	33.3	32.2	31.2	30.2	29.2	28.3	27.5	26.7
175	79.55		36.7	35.4	34.2	33.1	32.1	31.1	30.1	29.2	28.3	27.5
180	81.82		37.7	36.4	35.2	34.1	33.0	32.0	31.0	30.0	29.1	28.3
185	84.09		38.7	37.4	36.2	35.0	33.9	32.8	31.8	30.8	29.9	29.0
190	86.36		39.8	38.5	37.2	36.0	34.8	33.7	32.7	31.7	30.7	29.8
195	88.64		40.8	39.5	38.2	36.9	35.7	34.6	33.5	32.5	31.5	30.6
200	90.91		41.9	40.5	39.1	37.9	36.7	35.5	34.4	33.4	32.3	31.4
205	93.18		42.9	41.5	40.1	38.8	37.6	36.4	35.3	34.2	33.2	32.2
210	95.45		44.0	42.5	41.1	39.8	38.5	37.3	36.1	35.0	34.0	33.0
215	97.73		45.0	43.5	42.1	40.7	39.4	38.2	37.0	35.9	34.8	33.7
220	100.00		46.1	44.5	43.1	41.7	40.3	39.1	37.8	36.7	35.6	34.5
225	102.27		47.1	45.5	44.0	42.6	41.2	39.9	38.7	37.5	36.4	35.3
230	104.55		48.2	46.6	45.0	43.5	42.2	40.8	39.6	38.4	37.2	36.1
235	106.82		49.2	47.6	46.0	44.5	43.1	41.7	40.4	39.2	38.0	36.9
240	109.09		50.3	48.6	47.0	45.4	44.0	42.6	41.3	40.0	38.8	37.7
245	111.36		51.3	49.6	47.9	46.4	44.9	43.5	42.1	40.9	39.6	38.5
250	113.64		52.4	50.6	48.9	47.3	45.8	44.4	43.0	41.7	40.4	39.2
255	115.91		53.4	51.6	49.9	48.3	46.7	45.3	43.9	42.5	41.2	40.0
260	118.18		54.5	52.6	50.9	49.2	47.7	46.2	44.7	43.4	42.1	40.8
265	120.45		55.5	53.6	51.9	50.2	48.6	47.0	45.6	44.2	42.9	41.6
270	122.73		56.5	54.6	52.8	51.1	49.5	47.9	46.4	45.0	43.7	42.4
275	125.00		57.6	55.7	53.8	52.1	50.4	48.8	47.3	45.9	44.5	43.2
280	127.27		58.6	56.7	54.8	53.0	51.3	49.7	48.2	46.7	45.3	43.9
285	129.55		59.7	57.7	55.8	54.0	52.2	50.6	49.0	47.5	46.1	44.7
290	131.82		60.7	58.7	56.8	54.9	53.2	51.5	49.9	48.4	46.9	45.5
295	134.09		61.8	59.7	57.7	55.9	54.1	52.4	50.7	49.2	47.7	46.3
300	136.36		62.8	60.7	58.7	56.8	55.0	53.3	51.6	50.0	48.5	47.1

Body Mass Index Chart (cont'd.)

5'8"	5'9"	5'10"	5'11"	6'	6'1"	6'2"	6'3"	6'4"	6'5"	6'6"	6'7"	6'8"
68	69	70	71	72	73	74	75	76	77	78	79	80
173	175	178	180	183	185	188	191	193	196	198	201	203
15.2	14.8	14.4	14.0	13.6	13.2	12.9	12.5	12.2	11.9	11.6	11.3	11.0
16.0	15.5	15.1	14.7	14.3	13.9	13.5	13.2	12.8	12.5	12.2	11.9	11.6
16.8	16.3	15.8	15.4	14.9	14.5	14.2	13.8	13.4	13.1	12.7	12.4	12.1
17.5	17.0	16.5	16.1	15.6	15.2	14.8	14.4	14.0	13.7	13.3	13.0	12.7
18.3	17.8	17.3	16.8	16.3	15.9	15.4	15.0	14.6	14.3	13.9	13.5	13.2
19.0	18.5	18.0	17.5	17.0	16.5	16.1	15.7	15.2	14.9	14.5	14.1	13.8
19.8	19.2	18.7	18.2	17.7	17.2	16.7	16.3	15.9	15.4	15.1	14.7	14.3
20.6	20.0	19.4	18.9	18.3	17.8	17.4	16.9	16.5	16.0	15.6	15.2	14.9
21.3	20.7	20.1	19.6	19.0	18.5	18.0	17.5	17.1	16.6	16.2	15.8	15.4
22.1	21.5	20.8	20.3	19.7	19.2	18.7	18.2	17.7	17.2	16.8	16.4.	16.0
22.9	22.2	21.6	21.0	20.4	19.8	19.3	18.8	18.3	17.8	17.4	16.9	16.5
23.6	22.9	22.3	21.7	21.1	20.5	19.9	19.4	18.9	18.4	17.9	17.5	17.1
24.4	23.7	23.0	22.4	21.7	21.2	20.6	20.0	19.5	19.0	18.5	18.1	17.6
25.1	24.4	23.7	23.1	22.4	21.8	21.2	20.7	20.1	19.6	19.1	18.6	18.2
25.9	25.2	24.4	23.8	23.1	22.5	21.9	21.3	20.7	20.2	19.7	19.2	18.7
26.7	25.9	25.2	24.5	23.8	23.1	22.5	21.9	21.3	20.8	20.3	19.8	19.3
27.4	26.6	25.9	25.2	24.5	23.8	23.2	22.5	22.0	21.4	20.8	20.3	19.8
28.2	27.4	26.6	25.9	25.1	24.5	23.8	23.2	22.6	22.0	21.4	20.9	20.4
28.9	28.1	27.3	26.6	25.8	25.1	24.4	23.8	23.2	22.6	22.0	21.4	20.9
29.7	28.9	28.0	27.3	26.5	25.8	25.1	24.4	23.8	23.2	22.6	22.0	21.5
30.5	29.6	28.8	28.0	27.2	26.4	25.7	25.1	24.4	23.8	23.2	22.6	22.0
31.2	30.3	29.5	28.7	27.9	27.1	26.4	25.7	25.0	24.4	23.7	23.1	22.6
32.0	31.1	30.2	29.4	28.5	27.8	27.0	26.3	25.6	25.0	24.3	23.7	23.1
32.8	31.8	30.9	30.0	29.2	28.4	27.7	26.9	26.2	25.5	24.9	24.3	23.7
33.5	32.6	31.6	30.7	29.9	29.1	28.3	27.6	26.8	26.1	25.5	24.8	24.2
34.3	33.3	32.4	31.4	30.6	29.7	28.9	28.2	27.4	26.7	26.1	25.4	24.8
35.0	34.0	33.1	32.1	31.3	30.4	29.6	28.8	28.1	27.3	26.6	26.0	25.3
35.8	34.8	33.8	32.8	31.9	31.1	30.2	29.4	28.7	27.9	27.2	26.5	25.9
36.6	35.5	34.5	33.5	32.6	31.7	30.9	30.1	29.3	28.5	27.8	27.1	26.4
37.3	36.3	35.2	34.2	33.3	32.4	31.5	30.7	29.9	29.1	28.4	27.7	27.0
38.1	37.0	35.9	34.9	34.0	33.1	32.2	31.3	30.5	29.7	29.0	28.2	27.5
38.9	37.7	36.7	35.6	34.7	33.7	32.8	31.9	31.1	30.3	29.5	28.8	28.1
39.6	38.5	37.4	36.3	35.3	34.4	33.5	32.6	31.7	30.9	30.1	29.4	28.6
40.4	39.2	38.1	37.0	36.0	35.0	34.1	33.2	32.3	31.5	30.7	29.9	29.2
41.1	40.0	38.8	37.7	36.7	35.7	34.7	33.8	32.9	32.1	31.3	30.5	29.7
41.9	40.7	39.5	38.4	37.4	36.4	35.4	34.4	33.5	32.7	31.8	31.0	30.3
42.7	41.4	40.3	39.1	38.1	37.0	36.0	35.1	34.2	33.3	32.4	31.6	30.8
43.4	42.2	41.0	39.8	38.7	37.7	36.7	35.7	34.8	33.9	33.0	32.2	31.4
44.2	42.9	41.7	40.5	39.4	38.3	37.3	36.3	35.4	34.5	33.6	32.7	31.9
44.9	43.7	42.4	41.2	40.1	39.0	38.0	36.9	36.0	35.1	34.2	33.3	32.5
45.7	44.4	43.1	41.9	40.8	39.7	38.6	37.6	36.6	35.6	34.7	33.9	33.0

If your weight or height are not on this chart, you can calculate your own BMI with this formula:

$$BMI = \frac{\text{Weight in pounds} \times 704}{(\text{Height in inches})^2}$$

If you prefer the metric system, the formula looks like this:

$$BMI = \frac{\text{Weight in kilograms}}{(\text{Height in meters})^2}$$

Based on research conducted in large numbers of people, we believe the most desirable BMI is below 25 and ideally as low as 20. By any estimate, a BMI of 30 or above puts you at a higher risk for disease. Although some people will never be able to attain the optimal BMI, a more modest goal of dropping 1 or 2 BMI units can make a big difference to your health.

Date   _____

Height   _____

Weight   _____

Cholesterol count   _____

HDL count   _____

Triglyceride count   _____

Blood pressure   _____

Waist measurement   _____

Hip measurement   _____

Waist-to-Hip Ratio   _____

Body Mass Index   _____

II. PERSONAL WEIGHT HISTORY

It is very useful to understand the origins of your weight problem and the history of your dieting experiences. By examining past practices and patterns, you will be better able to avoid pitfalls that have caused you to abandon diets in the past. In this section, you can also set realistic goals for yourself and record the calorie count you'll need to get there.

Have I been struggling with weight control all my life? Or is this a problem of relatively recent origin? _____

_____

Did my weight problems begin with puberty, pregnancy, menopause, or some other momentous physiological event?

_____

_____

Did I experience any extreme trauma, such as sexual abuse, that may be linked to my weight gain? _____

_____

Is my weight problem linked to lifestyle and stress? Or are more complex psychological issues involved? _____

_____

The main reasons I want to lose weight are _____

_____

The highest adult weight I have reached is _____

The lowest adult weight I have maintained for a year is _____

What kind of weight loss have I been able to maintain in the past? _____

_____

What kind of weight loss has resulted in almost immediate regain? _____

_____

My long-range weight goal is _____

In the next year, my weight goal is _____

    I need a diet of _____ calories in order to lose 10 percent of my weight. (Guidelines for making these calculations are presented in Chapter 8.)

    When I am ready to lose another 10 percent of my weight, I will need a diet of _____ calories.

III. THE FOOD DIARY

Most overweight people vastly underestimate the amount of food they eat, sometimes by as much as 75 percent. That's why I believe it is almost impossible to control your weight without a food diary. A good diary tells you exactly what you are eating, why, and when. Think of it as an X-ray of your food habits.

    When you first begin the Getting Healthy program, I recommend that you maintain a diary faithfully for at least one month (and preferably longer) to gain a clear, detailed snapshot of your eating patterns. As you accumulate entries, you'll gather a wealth of information about how you eat and patterns will begin to emerge. Once your weight control program becomes routine, you can loosen up a bit, but it is a good habit to continue making notations several days a week. It is also an excellent tool for getting back on track if you lapse from time to time.

    Here are some other pointers:

Always carry the diary with you.
Don't say you're going to write something down later—take the notebook out immediately after you have eaten and make your entries. If you don't want to do this in public, excuse yourself for a moment. If you try to make an educated guess long after a meal is over, chances are you will understate what you have actually eaten. Over time, that can amount to a lot of extra calories.

Include everything you eat and drink.
Write down everything that goes into your mouth, including water, the butter on your bread, the chips before dinner, even the mints as you leave a restaurant. At a minimum, a diary entry should include the following information:

- ❖ What you ate
- ❖ What time you ate
- ❖ What else you were doing

It is time-consuming to record your calories, but it is also very important. If you are using Getting Healthy menu plans, calorie counts are provided. If you are improvising with menus of your own, purchase an inexpensive calorie counter at your local bookstore and make the calculations on the spot.

Be aware of your moods.
When possible, include at least a brief note describing your mood when you ate. If you have time, more elaborate comments are valuable. For example, you might try to answer at least some of the following questions at every meal:

- ❖ Why did I eat this?
- ❖ How did I feel when I ate this?
- ❖ Could I have chosen a healthier food?
- ❖ Did I eat because I was hungry?

Review your food diary regularly.
Use your diary as a blueprint for improvement. If you discover a certain time when you are always hungry—late in the evening or in the mid-afternoon—plan for a meal or a snack. If you are

eating high-fat foods because they're readily available, look for ways to create an alternative—for example, you might bring lunch to work instead of buying it at the employee cafeteria.

As you analyze your diary, look for triggers that may lead to overeating. Ask yourself:

❖ Do I eat a lot after dinner?

❖ Do I snack too often?

❖ Do I eat more at family or business settings?

❖ Am I eating because I am hungry or because food has a calming effect on me?

❖ Was this meal an appropriate part of my weight control program?

❖ Am I in control?

Here is a food diary format designed to make this routine as easy as possible:

Food/Calories   _____   _____

                 _____   _____

                 _____   _____

                 _____   _____

Date/Time   _____

Place   _____

Mood   _____

Comments   _____

A typical entry might read:

Food	½ cup fresh fruit	60 calories
	1 cup oatmeal	160 calories
	½ cup whole milk	75 calories
	Coffee with one-percent milk	—

Date/Time	Wednesday, Sept. 12/Breakfast, 7 A.M.	
Place	Home	
Mood	Tired from lack of sleep	

Another example:

Food	Salad	25 calories
	Small steak	165 calories
	Grilled vegetables	50 calories
	1 slice bread with butter	180 calories
	Two glasses of wine	180 calories
	Piece of carrot cake	550 calories
Date/Time	Thursday, Sept. 20/Dinner, 8 P.M.	
Place	Marlin's bar and grill	
Mood	Tense business dinner with boss	
Comments	Didn't really want to order the second glass of wine or the dessert but felt social pressure to join boss	

IV. EXERCISE LOG

Good exercise habits are as important to successful weight control as good eating habits. Keeping an exercise log allows you to monitor your routine and keep an eye out for obstacles and barriers. For example, you may discover that it is harder for you to exercise regularly under stress, even though you might benefit most from it at this time. You may also be able to identify revealing correlations between your eating and exercise habits.

In the first part of your log, you should spell out your goals:

My baseline fitness level (use results from the one-mile timed walk, Chapter 15) is_____ .

I plan to exercise _____ days a week.

Every day I will devote _____ minutes to aerobic exercise and every other day I will do _____ minutes of resistance exercises.

The time of day that is generally best for me to exercise is

_____ .

I will exercise _____ (at home, at the health club, in the park, etc.).

The equipment I will need is _____

_____ .

These are the exercises I will do:

_____

_____

_____

Once you have spelled out your objectives, you can use the log sheets on the pages that follow and record the exercises you do every day.

—————————— ❖ ❖ ❖ ——————————

STRETCHES FOR AEROBIC EXERCISES

Date _____

Stretches	Check When Completed
Standing hamstring	☐
Standing bent-knee hamstring	☐
Seated two-leg hamstring	☐
Seated one-leg hamstring	☐
Supine hamstring	☐
Quadriceps	☐
Prone quadriceps	☐
Calf	☐
Single knee hug	☐
Double knee hug	☐
Knee crossover	☐
Groin	☐
Back-arch stretch	☐
Lower-torso stretch	☐

— ❖ ❖ ❖ —

AEROBIC WALKING PROGRAM

Date _____

| Walking | Warm-up | Distance | Cooldown |

Date _____

| Walking | Warm-up | Distance | Cooldown |

Date _____

| Walking | Warm-up | Distance | Cooldown |

Date _____

| Walking | Warm-up | Distance | Cooldown |

— ❖ ❖ ❖ —

STRETCHES FOR RESISTANCE EXERCISES

Date

Stretches	**Check When Completed**
Shoulder shrug	☐
Neck stretch	☐
Side stretch	☐
Behind-the-back stretch	☐
Overhead stretch	☐
Behind-the-back stretch with towel	☐
Overhead stretch with towel	☐
Standing upper back	☐
Behind-the-head triceps	☐
Cross-face deltoid	☐
Standing latissimus/arms folded	☐
Twist	☐
Supine overhead	☐

— ❖ ❖ ❖ —

RESISTANCE EXERCISES

Date _____

Exercise		Number of Sets
Abdominals	Floor crunches	_____
	Curl crunches	_____
	Knee-ups	_____
	Cross twists	_____
	Flat cross twists	_____
	Pelvic tilt	_____
Pushes	Wall pushes	_____
	Counter pushes	_____
	Knee pushes	_____
	Push-ups	_____
Hips and Buttocks	External rotations	_____
	Three-angle leg raises	_____
Back	Windmills	_____
Rubber Band Exercises	Butterfly	_____
	Bow and arrow	_____
	Standing row	_____
	Seated cable row	_____
	Biceps curl	_____
Weights	Overhead press	_____
	Lateral raise	_____
	Front raise	_____
	Triceps kickbacks	_____
	Arm circles	_____
	Punches	_____
	Triceps overhead extension	_____

V. SPECIAL MOMENTS

You should also use your Weight Control Journal to highlight your triumphs. I urge you to make detailed and informative entries as often as possible—they are a marvelous record of your dieting experience.

These are examples of entries you might make:

"Today I felt satisfied with my meal plans and did not crave anything else. First time since I started!"

"Got urge for potato chips. Took a brief walk instead and then rewarded myself with two low-fat crackers."

"Ordered just what I had planned in the Chinese restaurant tonight. Everyone else was ordering spare ribs, but I asked for soup. It was delicious!"

Date _____

Experience _____

Date _____

Experience _____

Date _____

Experience _____

Date _____

Experience _____

Date _____

Experience _____

Date _____

Experience _____

Date _____

Experience _____

8

STRUCTURING
YOUR DIET

Let's say you are 5 feet, 5 inches tall, and weigh 175 pounds. Your goal is to lose 20 percent of your total body weight to bring yourself down to about 140 pounds. When you finally say, "This is it—the weight has got to come off," you may be tempted to embark on a severely restricted diet of, say, fewer than 1,000 calories a day in order to drop the pounds quickly. But extremely low-calorie diets require careful medical supervision, and faddish diets just don't work for most people.

WHY FAD DIETS DON'T WORK

Fad diets are often counterproductive because:

- ❖ They can leave you feeling irritable and deprived.
- ❖ They can slow down your metabolism so that your body burns fewer calories.
- ❖ They often depend almost exclusively on sheer willpower. Because it is hard to be disciplined when you feel hungry, weak, and tired, your risk of failure is higher.

❖ They seldom emphasize behavioral changes or the impor-
    tance of exercise, making it unlikely that you will be able
    to control your weight over time.

The Getting Healthy plan, by contrast, avoids the pain, frustration, and hunger characteristic of drastic diets and teaches
you the art of weight control for a lifetime. From Day One, you
are on the maintenance diet you can use forever.

HOW MUCH WEIGHT CAN YOU LOSE?

There is no way to know exactly how thin you can be. The lowest weight possible for you depends partly on your self-determi-
nation and self-discipline and partly on your metabolic capacity.
One of the most dramatic examples of how different people
respond to food comes from a study conducted by Eric
Ravussin, Ph.D., an obesity researcher at the National Institutes
of Health, who measured the energy expenditures of a group of
men over a twenty-four-hour period. In general, the more a man
weighed, the higher his metabolic rate, but there was tremendous variation. For example, two of the study subjects had the
same metabolic rate, yet incredibly, one weighed 150 pounds
and the other tipped the scales at 325 pounds. Although this
example is extreme, it illustrates how hard it is to predict the
body's physiological capabilities.

We do know that most people find it extremely difficult to
bring their weight below the lowest weight they have maintained
for a year as an adult. Even that can be difficult to reach if you
have been adding pounds steadily because your weight set point
seems continually to readjust itself upward.

To estimate your potential for weight loss, I use the guide-
lines developed by Thomas Wadden, Ph.D., director of the
Weight and Eating Disorders Program in the Department of
Psychiatry at the University of Pennsylvania:

First, estimate the lowest weight you have been able to
maintain for a year as an adult.

Second, add 1 pound for each year that has passed since then.

That calculation gives most people a weight goal they can reasonably expect to attain. For example, if you are forty-one years old and your lowest adult weight was 135 pounds, last reached at the age of thirty, then your target weight is now 146: that is, 135 + 11 (1 pound for each year since you were thirty).

Calculating Calories: The First 10 Percent

Once you have a long-range weight goal in mind, the next step is to determine how many calories you can consume to achieve it. No matter what your present weight, your first goal should be to shed no more than 10 percent of your total body weight. When you reach that goal, give yourself time to adjust to that weight and then tackle further weight loss, if you like.

To lose 10 percent of your body weight, you need to reduce your current calorie consumption by about 25 percent. If your final goal is a 20-percent weight loss, you eventually have to slash calories by about 35 percent; a 30-percent weight loss means dropping your calorie level by 45 percent. By losing weight in stages, these cutbacks aren't nearly as difficult as they may sound.

You'll be using the Calories You Need chart (see illustration) and the Formula for Calculating Calories, described below. The formula is based on more than six years of nutritional studies conducted at Rockefeller University by Jules Hirsch, M.D., Rudolph Leibel, M.D., and Michael Rosenbaum, M.D., some of the nation's foremost obesity researchers, and is adapted from work published in the *New England Journal of Medicine* in March 1995. It was developed for sedentary people, but if you are very physically active, you may be able to consume some additional calories. These numbers are averages—some people may need fewer calories, others more, depending in part on activity levels.

The Calories You Need

Height inches	58	59	60	61	62	63	64	65	66	67	68
Weight cm	147	150	152	155	157	160	163	165	168	170	173
lb kg											
100.0 45.5	1848	1871	1894	1917	1939	1962	1985	2007	2029	2052	2074
105.0 47.7	1887	1910	1934	1957	1980	2003	2026	2049	2072	2095	2117
110.0 50.0	1924	1948	1972	1996	2020	2043	2067	2090	2113	2136	2160
115.0 52.3	1961	1985	2010	2034	2058	2082	2106	2130	2154	2177	2201
120.0 54.5	1997	2022	2046	2071	2096	2120	2145	2169	2193	2217	2241
125.0 56.8	2032	2057	2082	2107	2132	2157	2182	2207	2231	2256	2280
130.0 59.1	2066	2092	2117	2143	2168	2194	2219	2244	2269	2294	2318
135.0 61.4	2099	2125	2152	2177	2203	2229	2255	2280	2305	2331	2356
140.0 63.6	2132	2159	2185	2211	2238	2264	2290	2316	2341	2367	2393
145.0 65.9	2164	2191	2218	2245	2271	2298	2324	2350	2377	2403	2429
150.0 68.2	2195	2223	2250	2277	2304	2331	2358	2385	2411	2437	2464
155.0 70.5	2226	2254	2282	2309	2337	2364	2391	2418	2445	2472	2498
160.0 72.7	2257	2285	2313	2341	2368	2396	2423	2451	2478	2505	2532
165.0 75.0	2286	2315	2343	2371	2399	2427	2455	2483	2511	2538	2566
170.0 77.3	2315	2344	2373	2402	2430	2458	2487	2515	2543	2571	2598
175.0 79.5	2344	2373	2402	2431	2460	2489	2518	2546	2574	2603	2631
180.0 81.8	2372	2402	2431	2461	2490	2519	2548	2577	2605	2634	2662
185.0 84.1	2400	2430	2460	2489	2519	2548	2578	2607	2636	2665	2693
190.0 86.4	2427	2458	2488	2518	2548	2577	2607	2637	2666	2695	2724
195.0 88.6	2454	2485	2515	2546	2576	2606	2636	2666	2695	2725	2754
200.0 90.9	2481	2512	2543	2573	2604	2634	2665	2695	2725	2754	2784
205.0 93.2	2507	2538	2570	2601	2631	2662	2693	2723	2753	2784	2814
210.0 95.5	2533	2565	2596	2627	2658	2689	2720	2751	2782	2812	2843
215.0 97.7	2558	2590	2622	2654	2685	2716	2748	2779	2810	2840	2871
220.0 100.0	2584	2616	2648	2680	2712	2743	2775	2806	2837	2868	2899
225.0 102.3	2608	2641	2673	2705	2738	2769	2801	2833	2864	2896	2927
230.0 104.5	2633	2666	2698	2731	2763	2795	2828	2860	2891	2923	2955
235.0 106.8	2657	2690	2723	2756	2789	2821	2854	2886	2918	2950	2982
240.0 109.1	2681	2714	2748	2781	2814	2846	2879	2912	2944	2976	3009
245.0 111.4	2704	2738	2772	2805	2838	2872	2905	2937	2970	3003	3035
250.0 113.6	2728	2762	2796	2829	2863	2896	2930	2963	2996	3029	3061
255.0 115.9	2751	2785	2819	2853	2887	2921	2954	2988	3021	3054	3087
260.0 118.2	2774	2808	2843	2877	2911	2945	2979	3012	3046	3079	3113
265.0 120.5	2796	2831	2866	2900	2935	2969	3003	3037	3071	3104	3138
270.0 122.7	2818	2854	2889	2923	2958	2993	3027	3061	3095	3129	3163
275.0 125.0	2841	2876	2911	2946	2981	3016	3051	3085	3120	3154	3188
280.0 127.3	2862	2898	2934	2969	3004	3039	3074	3109	3143	3178	3212
285.0 129.5	2884	2920	2956	2991	3027	3062	3097	3132	3167	3202	3237
290.0 131.8	2905	2942	2978	3014	3049	3085	3120	3156	3191	3226	3261
295.0 134.1	2927	2963	2999	3036	3072	3107	3143	3179	3214	3249	3284
300.0 136.4	2948	2984	3021	3057	3094	3130	3166	3201	3237	3273	3308

The Calories You Need (cont'd.)

69	70	71	72	73	74	75	76	77	78	79	80
175	178	180	183	185	188	191	193	196	198	201	203
2096	2118	2140	2162	2183	2205	2226	2248	2269	2291	2312	2333
2140	2162	2185	2207	2229	2251	2273	2295	2317	2339	2360	2382
2183	2205	2228	2251	2274	2296	2319	2341	2363	2385	2408	2430
2224	2247	2271	2294	2317	2340	2363	2386	2408	2431	2453	2476
2265	2288	2312	2336	2359	2383	2406	2429	2452	2475	2498	2521
2304	2329	2353	2377	2400	2424	2448	2472	2495	2519	2542	2565
2343	2368	2392	2417	2441	2465	2489	2513	2537	2561	2585	2608
2381	2406	2431	2456	2480	2505	2529	2554	2578	2602	2626	2651
2418	2443	2469	2494	2519	2544	2569	2594	2618	2643	2667	2692
2454	2480	2506	2531	2557	2582	2607	2633	2658	2683	2707	2732
2490	2516	2542	2568	2594	2620	2645	2671	2696	2721	2747	2772
2525	2551	2578	2604	2630	2656	2682	2708	2734	2760	2785	2811
2559	2586	2613	2639	2666	2692	2719	2745	2771	2797	2823	2849
2593	2620	2647	2674	2701	2728	2755	2781	2808	2834	2860	2886
2626	2654	2681	2708	2736	2763	2790	2817	2843	2870	2897	2923
2659	2686	2714	2742	2769	2797	2824	2852	2879	2906	2933	2960
2691	2719	2747	2775	2803	2831	2858	2886	2913	2941	2968	2995
2722	2751	2779	2807	2836	2864	2892	2920	2947	2975	3003	3030
2753	2782	2811	2839	2868	2896	2925	2953	2981	3009	3037	3065
2784	2813	2842	2871	2900	2929	2957	2986	3014	3043	3071	3099
2814	2843	2873	2902	2931	2960	2989	3018	3047	3075	3104	3132
2844	2873	2903	2933	2962	2991	3021	3050	3079	3108	3137	3165
2873	2903	2933	2963	2993	3022	3052	3081	3111	3140	3169	3198
2902	2932	2962	2993	3023	3053	3083	3112	3142	3171	3201	3230
2930	2961	2992	3022	3052	3083	3113	3143	3173	3203	3232	3262
2958	2989	3020	3051	3082	3112	3143	3173	3203	3233	3263	3293
2986	3017	3049	3080	3111	3141	3172	3203	3233	3264	3294	3324
3013	3045	3077	3108	3139	3170	3201	3232	3263	3294	3324	3355
3041	3072	3104	3136	3167	3199	3230	3261	3292	3323	3354	3385
3067	3099	3132	3163	3195	3227	3258	3290	3321	3352	3384	3415
3094	3126	3159	3191	3223	3255	3287	3318	3350	3381	3413	3444
3120	3153	3185	3218	3250	3282	3314	3346	3378	3410	3442	3473
3146	3179	3212	3244	3277	3309	3342	3374	3406	3438	3470	3502
3171	3205	3238	3271	3304	3336	3369	3401	3434	3466	3498	3530
3197	3230	3264	3297	3330	3363	3396	3429	3461	3494	3526	3559
3222	3255	3289	3323	3356	3389	3422	3455	3488	3521	3554	3586
3246	3280	3314	3348	3382	3415	3449	3482	3515	3548	3581	3614
3271	3305	3339	3373	3407	3441	3475	3508	3542	3575	3608	3641
3295	3330	3364	3398	3433	3467	3501	3534	3568	3602	3635	3668
3319	3354	3389	3423	3458	3492	3526	3560	3594	3628	3661	3695
3343	3378	3413	3448	3482	3517	3551	3586	3620	3654	3688	3721

Once you've done these calculations, you will know how many calories you can eat every day, given your height and weight, to pursue the weight loss you want. Be sure to enter your caloric requirements in your Weight Control Journal.

Calculating Calories for Weight Loss

1. Refer to the place on The Calories You Need chart (see pages 110–111) where your height meets your weight. That's how many calories it takes to maintain your current weight.

   To maintain my current weight, my caloric requirement is _____

2. If your first goal is to lose 10 percent of your body weight, multiply the answer in step 1 by 0.75. That figure represents your new caloric requirement.

   My new daily caloric requirement is _____

Your Next Weight-Loss Goal

After you have shed 10 percent of your body weight, you will feel terrific, perhaps better than you have felt in a long time. Most likely, you will be getting positive reinforcement from friends and family: "You've lost weight!" "You look wonderful!" You may be tempted to keep up the momentum and immediately charge ahead by reducing your caloric intake even further.

Believe it or not, this is the time to take a break from dieting and let your body adjust. Ideally, you should keep your weight stable for at least three months before trying to lose additional pounds; at a minimum, wait one full month. Meanwhile, allow yourself to feel good about having accomplished your most important goal—reaching a healthier weight and greatly reducing the chances of serious illness. Remember, this isn't a race; it's an ongoing process. Be patient. Work with your body, but don't push too hard. Taking a little time off is the best way to allow your new metabolism level to stabilize.

Then, you can slowly begin to reduce again. A reasonable new goal is to lose another 10 percent of your original body weight. Remember, you are basing your new calculations on your original weight:

Take your answer from step 1 on the previous page.

Multiply it by 0.65.

That tells you how many calories you need to lose 20 percent of your original body weight.

You can continue to use this formula until you have achieved your final weight goal. For example, if you need to lose 30 percent of your body weight, multiply the answer in step 1 by 55 percent.

Need further clarification? The story of Alice illustrates these calculations.

An Example of Calorie Counting

Alice is 5 feet, 2 inches tall, weighs 220 pounds, and leads a very sedentary life. By consulting The Calories You Need chart, Alice discovers that she needs 2,712 calories daily to maintain her present weight. (By the way, you may find it easier to make your calculations by rounding up or down to the nearest 100 calories; for example, Alice could have based her calorie count on 2,700 calories a day.)

Step 1   Alice's food diary reveals that she is eating more than 2,712 calories a day, which means her weight is gradually creeping higher. She first accustoms herself to a 2,712-calorie diet to stop the gain.

Step 2   Alice's next goal is to lose 10 percent of her total body weight, or 22 pounds. To accomplish this, she decreases her calorie consumption by 25 percent:

$$2{,}712 \text{ calories} \times 0.75 = 2{,}034 \text{ calories}$$

Alice loses about 1 pound every week on a diet of about 2,034 calories and achieves her first goal in about five months.

Step 3   Having lost 10 percent of her total body weight, Alice waits for two months before cutting her calories further. During this time, she concentrates on refining her exercise regimen and reinforcing new food habits.

Step 4   When Alice feels ready to begin the next stage of reducing, she aims for another 10-percent weight loss (20 percent of her original body weight). To attain that goal, she cuts her original 2,712-calorie diet by 35 percent:

$$2,712 \text{ calories} \times 0.65 = 1,763$$

In approximately five more months, Alice reaches 176 pounds. Dropping from 2,712 calories to 1,763 in one step would have been more difficult, but Alice discovers that breaking the process into several smaller steps, with adjustment time in between, was not nearly so hard. Although she is still higher than her optimal weight, she is at a much healthier place than before.

Step 5   If Alice wants to lose even more weight—say a total weight loss of 30 percent—she will have to be extremely cautious. First, she must allow another period of adjustment. During that time, she should also pay careful attention to her current eating patterns and make sure her diet is balanced. After at least a month's pause, she can try again.

To lose a total of 30 percent of her original body weight, Alice will have to cut out 45 percent of her original calorie count.

$$2,712 \text{ calories} \times 0.55 = 1,492 \text{ calories}$$

Again, the slow approach works. If Alice had dropped immediately to 1,492 calories from 2,712, she might have found her diet too restrictive to tolerate over the long term. Reducing slowly allows her to reach her goals without feeling deprived.

AN APPROACH TO FOOD THAT WORKS

When you first begin my program, you may prefer to be told exactly what to eat—the fewer choices you have, the easier you may find it. The comprehensive menu plans in Part IV help you do just that.

- ❖ Menu Plan I is a low-fat, high-carbohydrate diet.
- ❖ Menu Plan II features more fibrous vegetables and fewer simple carbohydrates and starches in order to maintain a lower glycemic index.

As we understand more about insulin resistance and the importance of the glycemic index, we are beginning to understand why some people lose weight more readily on Menu Plan II. If you have any of the following medical conditions in your own or your family's history, Menu Plan II may be most effective for you: insulin resistance; diabetes; high triglycerides and a low HDL count; hypertension; or early atherosclerosis despite normal cholesterol levels.

Eventually, we will have more data on which to base our initial recommendations, but for now, I suggest you start with the high-carbohydrate diet and switch after two months if you have not achieved a weight loss of at least 4 pounds. I've given you two weeks of menus for each plan, followed by easy-to-use recipes for many of the dishes.

In the weight control community, we call these menu plans *stimulus narrowing,* which means limiting your food choices in order to reduce temptation. By keeping "dangerous" foods out of the house and following strict meal plans every day of the week, you lessen the risk of straying back to old habits. Stimulus narrowing is most effective when you are highly motivated but fearful of temptation.

In the long run, however, strict rules become stifling. Once a menu plan gets tedious, or doesn't include enough of the foods you really enjoy, it is natural to start looking for excuses to cheat. When you begin to rebel against structured menu plans, you need to know how to improvise. That's when the flexibility that is the hallmark of the Getting Healthy approach becomes most useful.

As you become more confident in your ability to lose weight, you can add more variety to your menu with food exchanges and ingredient substitutions. Almost everyone who successfully loses weight, and keeps it off, eventually learns how to make intelligent choices. You do not have to be deprived of foods that you adore to control your weight. There are ways to include almost everything you like in your diet, although your passion for high-fat or high-sugar foods can only be indulged in very small quantities. For some people, just a taste of a forbidden food satisfies the craving. For others, that is enough to throw the diet off balance. My philosophy is to encourage experimentation so that you can find out what works for you.

HOW WEIGHT COMES OFF

When you understand how your body sheds weight, it will become more apparent why pounds sometimes drop off like magic and other times refuse to budge.

Losing Water Weight

Water retention accounts for many of the short-term fluctuations you may experience in body weight. In the first few days of any diet, most people drop several pounds. I'm delighted if your spirits soar as a result, but the truth is, you are losing weight that will come right back as soon as you stop counting calories so rigorously.

According to a study conducted by Victor Katch, Ph.D., a professor in the Department of Exercise Science at the University of Massachusetts, the composition of weight loss changes over time so that you lose increasingly more fat and less water:

Stage 1   The first three days of a diet, weight loss is 70 percent water, 5 percent protein, and 25 percent fat.

Stage 2   Days 11 to 13 of a diet, weight loss is 19 percent water, 12 percent protein, and 69 percent fat.

Stage 3   Days 21 to 24 of a diet, weight loss is 15 percent protein and 85 percent fat.

Stage 4   After 24 days, weight loss stabilizes at 25 percent protein and 75 percent fat.

On the other hand, there are times when your body retains excess water. Many women gain a few pounds just before their menstrual period begins. Fluid retention can be a common side effect of other hormonal changes and of some medications. It also occurs if you consume too many calories, particularly carbohydrates. Don't let short-term weight changes disrupt a long-term commitment to healthy eating. And don't panic if you suddenly gain 5 pounds after a careless day—that is just water weight and it will come off as soon as you get back on track with your diet.

The Oreo Cookie Effect

Another important principle to understand is that some weight loss can be achieved with very modest dietary modifications. Here is what can happen when you stop eating just one Oreo cookie:

❖ An Oreo cookie has 50 calories. Multiply that figure by the number of days in a year:

$$50 \text{ calories} \times 365 \text{ days/year} = 18{,}250 \text{ extra calories/year}$$

❖ You have to reduce your food intake by 3,500 calories to lose 1 pound of weight. Divide 18,250 calories by 3,500.

$$18{,}250 \text{ calories}/3{,}500 \text{ calories} = 5.2 \text{ pounds/year}$$

Theoretically, at least, this means you can lose more than 5 pounds in a year just by eating one less cookie a day, assuming no other dietary or lifestyle changes. Cut two Oreos out of your diet and you can lose 10 pounds in a year.

That's the good news. But a word of warning: Adding one of those cookies every day may have the opposite result—you'll gain 5 pounds within a year.

I saw the Oreo cookie effect on a man I'll call Jim. Jim stopped at a convenience store for breakfast every morning and used to order coffee, juice, a donut, and a bagel with extra cream cheese. By substituting a piece of fruit for the donut, cutting out the juice, and using a very thin layer of cream cheese, he cut out 500 calories a day without feeling the least bit deprived. That may not sound like much, but a total of about 15,000 calories a month resulted in a weight loss of about 35 pounds with very little effort.

Surviving Plateaus

Finally, you need to understand weight-loss plateaus, which are a dieter's curse. Even the gradual weight loss you experience on the Getting Healthy plan levels off from time to time and that feels very frustrating. People commonly say to me, "I have lost 10 percent of my previous weight, but I still feel fat. And I just can't seem to lose anything more. What can I do?"

There are a number of reasons you may reach a plateau. After the concentrated effort required to lose weight initially, you may find it hard to retain focus. Or, your body may just need a break. My advice is generally to sit tight, maintain your current caloric intake, keep exercising, and pay strict attention to any sign that your weight is creeping back on. Chances are that after a period of adjustment, you will start shedding those pounds again. Don't push yourself too hard—if you do, you may become so discouraged that you gain back everything you worked so hard to lose. If you feel motivated, step up the pace of your exercise regimen to give your dieting efforts both a psychological and a physical boost.

Remember, a 10-percent weight loss makes a big difference to your health. If you are following my diet, exercise, and behavior guidelines religiously, yet your body keeps resisting further weight loss, perhaps you have already reached your healthiest weight. Although the urge to lose may remain strong, at some point you must accept your body as it is. Remember my motto: The most important reason to lose weight is to stay healthy. Chasing any other goal is a surefire road to frustration.

9

GETTING STARTED

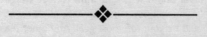

You are now armed with the background to succeed at the Getting Healthy plan. It helps to know what to expect in the first few days when you will probably experience the greatest discomfort. Despite the psychological lift that water-weight loss often provides, your system will likely experience a bit of a shock when you cut calories. Just thinking about the restrictions you have imposed can be enough to make you crave food. In this chapter, I'll talk about the timing of your commitment, what to anticipate, and how to manage your stress level.

TAKE THE READINESS TEST

Wait to begin my program until you can make a wholehearted commitment to it. Take this readiness test to see whether or not this is the right time for you to begin. If you can truthfully answer yes to the six questions here, you have a long-range and realistic view of weight loss and can start on the Getting Healthy program.

If there are one or two no's among your responses, you may not be ready. Try a two-week, no-regrets trial using my menu plans and exercises. If you discover this is a bad time to make a commitment, call it quits and come back when you feel ready. Meanwhile, just concentrate on keeping your weight stable.

Are you motivated?

It takes personal strength, determination, and commitment to stay with any menu plan, even a flexible one. Many times, I have seen people fail at weight control because they weren't fully committed to the rigors of changing lifelong habits. Make sure you have the energy to focus on weight control.

Are you clear about why you want to lose weight?

Most likely you will never be thin as a rail. Few of us are. Good health should be your foremost goal. Any other reason for wanting to lose weight—looking sexier, gaining the eye of someone special, feeling better about yourself—can also be valid, but in my view, preventing the illnesses associated with excess weight matters most. People who emphasize the association between weight and good health are most likely to stick with the program.

Are you prepared to start exercising?

Many sedentary people are intimidated by the idea of committing to an exercise program, but it can be a very gradual process. If you are a complete couch potato, all I ask is that you get started. Learn how to incorporate a little more movement in your daily life. As your body becomes accustomed to increased levels of physical activity, you will be able to exercise more vigorously.

Is this a good time to start?

Are there holidays, social occasions, or business gatherings coming up? Are you confident that you can deal with these situations? Or would it be better to wait until they are over? Ask yourself if you want to start your diet during the week or on the weekend. If you have already started a food diary, use it to identify activities associated with overeating and avoid starting your diet during one of these times.

Do you have a long-range view?

Don't impose false or arbitrary deadlines on yourself. Remember, your weight came on slowly and must be shed just as slowly if it is to stay off for good. Some people are initially motivated by a particular event—they want to lose weight for an upcoming wedding or an anniversary, for example. That's a reasonable goal, but once that event is over, it is important to set your sights on something new in order to stay on track.

Keeping your weight under control is an ongoing process, even after you have reached your goals. Although it is a lot easier to maintain a stable weight than to shed extra pounds, and much easier to sustain good habits than to break bad ones, you can't ever afford to let down your guard.

Are you willing to become an informed consumer?
Ultimately, I believe you will have to create your own diet. There is no way my menu plans and recipes can factor in your personal taste and the individual circumstances of your life. Lifetime weight control means developing an approach to food that works for *you*. Start the Getting Healthy program after you have cleared away any obstacles preventing you from concentrating on this new challenge.

PRACTICAL GUIDELINES THAT HELP

Once you decide you are ready, keep the following guidelines in mind.

Mentally prepare yourself for the first difficult days.
When you get started on a diet, the effort of remembering what you are and are not supposed to eat, how much, and when, will claim a lot of your energy. Eventually, it will become second nature to you, but for now, try to lighten up on your other commitments so that you can focus.

Take heart, knowing that a new routine will soon emerge. Within a few days, the initial discomfort of eating less fades. Your body will become accustomed to fewer calories and you may even feel newly energized. You may be amazed to discover how much less food you need to feel full.

Be optimistic.
A "can-do" outlook and a belief that you really can control your

weight generates enthusiasm, self-confidence, and a sense of accomplishment. If you've struggled and failed before, now is the time to break old habits, shed destructive feelings of help-lessness, and start anew. Repeat to yourself, "I am in control. I have the power to succeed at this diet." Reward yourself with enough positive messages, and gradually, you will internalize them and make them come true.

Be patient.

Remember our previous discussions of the feast-or-famine cycle? In the early days of a diet, your body senses a famine is coming and encourages you to look for food as a survival instinct. It takes great determination to resist this signal, but after a few days, the message to eat decreases and the process becomes a lot easier.

Be prepared for cravings.

At first, you may have an overwhelming desire to eat certain foods. A carbohydrate craving is most common because cutting back on sweets and starches means you are losing some of their medicating effect. Cravings gradually ease, but they may con-tinue to reappear from time to time. For example, many women experience strong cravings shortly before their menstrual period.

You may be able to satisfy cravings in small amounts. Eating a piece of fruit, a slice of bread, or a handful of pretzels adds less than 100 calories to your diet while quieting the message to eat carbohydrates. If you crave sweets, try a nonfat product, such as a graham cracker or a piece of sucking candy. If you can't cope without chocolate, see if three chocolate kisses will do the trick. Wait at least an hour before eating anything else to allow the craving to ease. Like medicine, a small dose of food may be ben-eficial, but a big dose has side effects—in this case, weight gain and perhaps an even greater craving.

Don't skip meals.

Your body needs to be refueled regularly, so it is very important not to miss a meal. Kathy Isoldi, one of the dietitians in my office, likes to tell her clients: "You wouldn't drive your car if the gas gauge was on empty, nor should you drive your body that way." If you want a snack at midday, enjoy a healthy one. If you overindulge at one meal—and almost everyone does from time to time—don't skip the next meal. Likewise, don't deliberately miss a meal in order to overeat later. Establish consistent habits and stick to them.

Have compassion for yourself.
All of us talk to ourselves, but unfortunately, the conversation we have is often negative: "I was wrong to do that." "I let myself down." People who are overweight often hear an especially cruel inner voice that says, "I'm fat. I have no control. I was born to suffer like this."

Stop it! One of your first tasks on the Getting Healthy program is to turn those negative messages around. I want you to start saying something entirely different to yourself. Try something like this:

> "I ate just what I had planned to eat today. I did a really great job."

> "I didn't need that second helping of potatoes. Well, most people go off track occasionally. I'm going to concentrate on doing better next time."

> "This problem is not entirely my fault. I'm fighting a heroic battle against a chronic medical condition."

When you begin to believe that you deserve compassion, support, and understanding, you'll find that your confidence and personal power will begin to grow. You are working hard and making a lot of sacrifices. Give yourself some credit. Don't punish yourself when you fall short of your own expectations. Do praise yourself for trying to improve your life.

Listen to your body.
When you first start to diet, you may have a mild, periodic headache or you may feel lightheaded or dizzy. Sometimes these feelings are related to water loss and can be relieved with a salty snack, such as a pickle or a cup of bouillon. Mild hunger pangs can often be satisfied with a piece of fruit or low-fat yogurt, at

only a small calorie count. Maintain an even flow of calories throughout the day and be sure you have not cut your calorie consumption below 1,200. If feelings of dizziness persist for more than a day or two, consult your doctor.

Stay off the scale.
Don't get on the scale for at least four weeks after beginning the Getting Healthy plan. Until then, focus on establishing a new routine and developing a sense of competence and well-being. When you do climb back on the scale, don't expect a weight loss of more than 2 pounds. The downfall of most dieters is a quest for quick, dramatic results.

Be flexible.
If you are overly strict when you start dieting, you may find it impossible to sustain the habit over time. Sometimes, it is appropriate to set aside your weight-loss goals. During the holidays, for example, it may be wise not to work too hard to lose weight. Concentrate, instead, on not gaining any new weight. If you get through the end-of-the-year holidays without putting on extra pounds, consider that enough of an accomplishment. A recent survey showed that the average person gains 4 pounds between Thanksgiving and New Year's Day—avoid that trap and you deserve a big pat on the back.

Also, you should not look at a moment of weakness (such as eating a large meal followed by a big dessert) as proof that you have failed or as an excuse to abandon your diet altogether. Instead, consider that slip a reminder to be vigilant. Think of all the days you did not lapse back to old patterns. Celebrate the moments you resisted temptation. Believe in your ability to win at weight control.

LEARNING TO MANAGE STRESS

Everyone knows what stress is, but few people realize how it contributes to weight control problems. Whether the source is family pressure, work expectations, or even a happy occasion, such as buying a house or getting married, stress directly affects the way you eat. You may be eating to celebrate or eating to console yourself—either way, you eat too much and weight piles on. Dieting itself can also become a source of stress.

Your ability to relax, especially in the first and toughest days of a diet, will help determine success. Although it is hard to eliminate stress altogether, there are ways to identify it, reduce it, and manage it. We all know examples in which two people have the same experience yet react to it in entirely different ways. One person can view job loss as catastrophic whereas someone else can consider it an opportunity. Although you can't control every event in your life, you may be able to change your reactions. For some people, reducing stress is almost like taking a diet pill—it actually suppresses the appetite by decreasing the level of certain compounds in the body that contribute to weight gain.

A good place to start is to learn what triggers stress. Let's say you're going out to dinner with business associates. Your typical response might be to order drinks and appetizers right away to relieve your own anxiety and to encourage everyone to relax. That is a knee-jerk reaction: Face stress, eat food, and drink alcohol. By practicing the stress-reduction techniques here, you can find ways to avoid this automatic impulse.

Identify stress-busting techniques that work for you.
Many people develop their own stress-busters. Regular exercise is one approach that works well. Exercise releases tension and over time it actually changes your physiology so that you are better able to handle stress. Carving out twenty minutes a day to listen to music or read a book is another technique that may work well for you. Do something special for yourself every day.

Isolate and release tension spots.
Everyone has especially sensitive spots where most of their tension tends to concentrate. The usual culprits are the neck, shoulders, jaw, lower back, and fists. To release some of this tension, tighten each muscle group as tautly as possible and then release it completely. Repeat this exercise several times, each time saying softly to yourself: "Tighten and release. Tighten and release."

You can do this exercise anywhere—at your desk, at home, even walking down the street. You'll be amazed at how much, and how quickly, it can help.

Practice deep breathing.
Deep breathing is another easy-to-do exercise. Breathe deeply through your nose three times in a row, exhaling forcibly through your mouth after each breath. To make sure you are breathing from your abdomen, rather than from the chest, place one hand in each place. Your chest should be almost still while you should be able to feel your abdomen moving with every breath. As you exhale, visualize yourself letting go of pent-up stress.

Learn to meditate.
This simple meditation technique takes about six minutes—not a huge time investment—yet the results are amazing. Many of the people I work with tell me they gain new energy and lose their urge to overeat. The more often you do this, the better you'll get at it.

Sit comfortably on a chair, in a quiet place where you will not be interrupted. Uncross your legs and rest your arms at your side. You should have nothing on your lap.

As you hear the instructions that follow, repeat one word silently to yourself as a kind of mantra. You might say, "relax," over and over again. The choice of words is up to you, but the goal is to keep your mind as focused and as still as possible.

You can have someone read these instructions to you slowly and softly or you can record them on tape yourself. The reader should keep an even, relaxed tone and pause at the end of every line:

Close your eyes and breathe deeply through your nose.

Exhale, slowly, through your mouth.

Breathe, slowly, through your nose.

Exhale slowly through your mouth.

And again.

Inhale.

Exhale.

And again.

As you continue to breathe, focus your attention on your head.

Feel your scalp relax.

Feel your face muscles loosen up.

Let your jaw drop slightly.

Continue to breathe deeply.

In and out.

In and out.

Now, relax your neck.

Feel the tension releasing from your shoulders.

Breathe in.

And out.

Feel your arms relax.

Feel your hands relax.

Feel the tension flowing out through your fingers.

Breathe in.

And out.

Let your body be supported by the chair.

Sink into the chair.

Feel the tension flowing out through your lower back.

Feel your legs relax.

Feel the tension flowing out through your feet and toes.

Sink into the chair.

Breathe in.

And out.

Relax.

Relax.

Feel your whole body relax.

Just sink into the chair.

Relax.

While you're in this deeply relaxed state, take a moment to reaffirm a positive message. You may want to say something about food or remind yourself of the good things in your life, of the people who love you, and of all you have to be thankful for. You might say:

"I am in charge of my self and my body."

"I choose what I want to eat and when."

"I can succeed in accomplishing my goals."

"There are many people who want to help me succeed."

After you have relaxed for a few minutes, count backward slowly from five to prepare yourself to emerge from the meditative state. Open your eyes, but don't move yet. Reorient yourself to the room. Get up slowly and give yourself a few minutes to get back into gear.

10

WEIGHT CONTROL
FOR A LIFETIME

Most people who lose significant amounts of weight end up regaining it within five years. We are trying to learn more about this. The newly discovered *ob* gene may play a role here, possibly by decreasing production of leptin, the fat-regulating hormone, so that over time, your metabolic rate decreases, your appetite increases, and you return to your original weight. That's why I'm so excited about the promise of leptin therapy.

Your approach to dieting may also be a culprit. I have seen many people lose weight too quickly, neglect their exercise, and ignore the lifestyle changes that are necessary to maintain a healthy weight for a lifetime. Inevitably, the weight comes back on.

The Getting Healthy experience is designed to address both the physiological and behavioral causes of weight gain. Because you learn healthy habits from the first pound you lose, you won't need to shift to a maintenance program once you reach your target weight. You may be able to eat a greater variety of foods and to increase your caloric intake, but basically the plan you have been following is the plan you will keep.

But there will still be some challenges ahead. If you have a tendency to put on weight, you will always have to be vigilant. Your body's natural desire to store fat remains a lifetime companion. You will always have to monitor your eating behavior, avoid high-fat and high-sugar foods, and exercise regularly, even if pharmaceutical treatments are successfuly developed. You will never be able to live and eat the way you once did. The hard work of maintaining a healthy weight is a lifelong project.

SURVIVING THE INEVITABLE LAPSE

Of course, staying on course sounds easier than it is. Sooner or later, you are going to stray from your diet. It happens to everyone. The key to controlling your weight for a lifetime is not to kick yourself when you become careless, but to understand what triggers a lapse and to learn to deal with it.

Three Reasons Why You Lapse

I often draw on the work of two respected psychologists to explain food lapses: G. Alan Marlatt, Ph.D., the director of Addictive Behaviors Research Center at the University of Washington in Seattle; and Judith R. Gordon, Ph.D., who is in private practice in Seattle. These psychologists have identified three common reasons for food lapses:

1. **Negative emotional states.** You lose control over the foods you eat because you feel anxious, depressed, bored, or lonely.

2. **Interpersonal conflicts.** You become careless after clashing with a spouse or some other family member, friend, or colleague.

3. **Social pressure.** You binge when you are in a social setting that makes you feel vulnerable or that reminds you of an earlier eating problem.

I have also noticed that some people lapse into old patterns months after ending a diet. This tends to happen at a moment when you finally recognize, deep down, that old habits are gone for good. Never again can you eat with careless abandon. Never again will you be able to enjoy a regular diet of high-fat, high-calorie food. From now on, you will always have to be vigilant if you are going to maintain an upper hand over your genetic and metabolic tendencies to gain weight. This reality can strike hard and it may spark a rebellion that takes the form of overeating.

Food lapses also trigger a physiological reaction that makes it hard to return to a healthy diet. Say you have eaten twice your usual allotment of calories for several days, which is not difficult to do with a couple of extra helpings of meat, fatty food, and sweets. Your body reacts as if you have suddenly rocked a steady boat—in a sense, everything that had been moving smoothly begins to swing wildly. The feast-or-famine response kicks in. The brain receives a message that says, "There is food out there somewhere. It is time to stock up."

If you weigh yourself after a careless week, you will probably see a gain of several pounds. That comes mostly from water retention, but it can be discouraging enough to lead to further overeating. And changes in your insulin, in other hormonal levels, and in your brain chemistry fuel hunger, worsening the challenge you face.

What's to be done? You may be tempted to toss all caution to the wind. Having lapsed once, you may feel that you will never get back your former discipline. Nonsense. Here are some rules to follow instead.

Overcoming Lapses

❖ **Don't despair.**   Overeating for a few days does not mean your whole diet has been trashed. The danger, as Kelly Brownell, Ph.D., director of the Yale Center for Eating and Weight Disorders, says, is that, "Lapse becomes relapse and then collapse."

❖ **Figure out why the lapse occurred.**   This is a perfect occasion to put your Weight Control Journal to work. If you have kept honest records, you will have a snapshot of recent events. Think about the moods and activities that may have contributed to falling off your diet. Chances are you will encounter similar situations again. Think about how you might deal with them differently next time.

❖ **Don't beat yourself up.**   What's done is done and the damage isn't irreversible. It may be helpful to confide in a friend or a counselor to talk through your evolving feelings toward food. Then stop focusing on your errors and move on with your life.

❖ **Get back on track.**   Don't overcompensate for the lapse by eating less; that will only tilt your system further askew. Start eating balanced meals again, knowing that a period of hunger often follows overindulgence—but will eventually fade once your body becomes reaccustomed to healthy food habits.

❖ **Keep in touch with the Getting Healthy program.**   If you were able to lose weight successfully with this book, you should refer to it from time to time, especially when your discipline is wavering. If you seem to be on a downward slope, you may want to return to my menu plans.

❖ **Feel like a winner.**   Every day that you successfully control your weight is a day of victory. Every day you maintain your new weight is a successful day. And every time you lapse, think of it as an opportunity to identify another obstacle in your life so that you can remove it.

❖ **Don't give up.**   You've come too far to go backward now. You have already proven your strength and determination. You have reason to feel proud. You are well on the way to getting healthy.

MISSION: LIFETIME WEIGHT CONTROL

Five other guidelines will help you keep weight off for good:

1. Let go of dieting.
2. Eat the foods you love—occasionally.
3. Don't panic if you gain back a few pounds.
4. Beware of the three-year rebound.
5. Enjoy your sense of control.

Let Go of Dieting

When healthy eating and exercise habits become more integrated into your life, you will begin to devote less attention to your weight problem. However, emerging from a long period of dieting into a normal relationship with food can be difficult. After focusing on weight loss for so long, you may experience an absence of purpose. You may find yourself at loose ends, unsure of what to do next. You may long for the positive feedback you got from friends and family as the pounds were melting away. You may actually begin to miss dieting itself.

I suggest that you try to find new hobbies or other activities to replace your fixation with food and weight. Perhaps now is the time to join a reading circle, take up a new sport, or become involved in a community project. Keep yourself busy, but don't forget to take time out to enjoy your freedom from weight obsession. After all, you have earned it.

Eat the Foods You Love—Occasionally

Many people who have been overweight in the past are afraid to eat once-favorite foods, especially if they are very rich in fats or sugars. If you deny yourself something you really want, however, you build up a reservoir of desire and the dam might burst out of control at a party or late one night at home. Instead of saying "no" to favored foods altogether, control your body's demands by giving into them from time to time. Once you have reached your healthiest weight, you can indulge your cravings occasionally—say, once a month, confident that you have the willpower to splurge without going overboard.

When it is time for your treat, enjoy yourself. Celebrate the special occasion. Plan to eat with a friend, in a public place. You don't need to feel the guilt that used to accompany these indulgences. You've earned this pleasure.

Don't Panic If You Gain Back a Few Pounds

Everyone gains back a little weight at some point soon after reaching the weight goal. Don't get upset. Often it is a sign that you are adjusting to real-world realities and no longer need to pay such strict attention to what you eat. If your weight stabilizes after you gain a few pounds, you have nothing to be concerned about. However, keep a careful eye on the situation and make sure it doesn't spiral out of control.

Beware of the Regain Risk

For reasons that physicians don't entirely understand, many people begin to put on pounds between 18 months and three years after a major weight loss. Although scientists are investigating metabolic explanations, the weight gain may simply be the result of a gradual return to old habits. You may be consuming more calories than you realize or perhaps you have become careless about your exercise routines. Perhaps you sustained an injury and got out of the exercise habit. It is easy to lose focus after a few years, and if you do, the pounds will gradually creep back on.

It is important to steady this sort of gain. When you feel your waist start to thicken, go back to the earlier chapters of this book and use the tools and strategies that worked best for you. Reread the material at the beginning of this chapter about surviving lapses. Use your food diary more often. Start counting calories again. Make sure you're getting enough exercise, which is the most potent tool we have for maintaining weight. Seek help from a friend, a counselor, or a physician if you feel it would be useful. Catch the problem early and you'll be able to get back on track painlessly.

Enjoy Your Sense of Control

Nothing tastes better than the feeling of being in control. Hopefully, you will be able to carry this sense of accomplishment to other areas of your life. After succeeding at weight control, many people find that their personal and professional lives function more smoothly. Bolstered by one success, you may be able to approach other challenges with equal determination and discipline. Typically, I hear people say, "I have beaten the toughest problem of all: controlling my weight. Surely, I can beat this problem, too."

PART FOUR

TWO MENU PLANS THAT WORK

◆ ◆ ◆

11

MENU PLAN I: THE LOW-FAT, HIGH-CARBOHYDRATE APPROACH

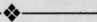

Menu Plan I is a low-fat, high-carbohydrate approach to losing weight. The balanced and nourishing meals feature chicken, fish, pasta, rice, potatoes, and a substantial variety of fruits and vegetables. Low-calorie snacks prevent you from feeling deprived or hungry. Combined with the system of food exchanges and ingredient substitutions I'll explain in Chapter 14, you should have the information you need to eat well while getting healthy. Although these menu plans have all the vitamins and minerals a healthy person should need, I have no objection if you want to take a multivitamin as extra insurance.

The menu plans here are structured for diets of approximately 1,200, 1,500, and 1,800 calories. Refer to Chapter 8 for a refresher course in determining how many calories you need to reach your weight goal. If the charts suggest you can consume more than 1,800 calories, you can increase food portions and add snacks. And if the right calorie count for you falls between the menu plans provided here, you can add some extra calories to customize the programs to your needs. Adding more vegetables and fruits to your diet is generally the healthiest way to increase the calorie count.

As we get started, let me again say thanks to Janet Feinstein, M.S., R.D., and Kathy Isoldi, M.S., R.D., the dietitians in my office, who designed Menu Plans I and II, calculated the food composition and calories so carefully, and tested the recipes in Chapter 13.

The approximate composition of each Getting Healthy high-carbohydrate diet is listed below. Some meals differ slightly in composition and calorie count, and I've rounded off some of the calculations to make the menus easier to use. There has been no compromise in terms of taste or nutritional value, however, and all of the meals are well balanced and low in fat.

1,200 calories
6 servings of protein
5 servings of starch
2 servings of milk
4 servings of vegetables
3 servings of fruit
1 serving of fat

In the 1,200-calorie high-carbohydrate diet, approximately 17 percent of your calories come from fat, 27 percent from protein, and 56 percent from carbohydrates.

1,500 calories
7 servings of protein
7 servings of starch
2 servings of milk
4 servings of vegetables
4 servings of fruit
2 servings of fat

In the 1,500-calorie high-carbohydrate diet, approximately 20 percent of your calories come from fat, 24 percent from protein, and 56 percent from carbohydrates.

1,800 calories
8 servings of protein
8 servings of starch
2 servings of milk
5 servings of vegetables
5 servings of fruit
3 servings of fat

In the 1,800-calorie high-carbohydrate diet, approximately 20 percent of your calories come from fat, 24 percent from protein, and 56 percent from carbohydrates.

A Few Words About Servings

Servings, or exchanges, represent an estimate of the number of calories in a given portion size or weight of a food. We have used them to make it easy to "exchange" between similar foods in order to add flexibility to your diet. For example, one-half cup of cooked pasta, peas, or corn have about the same number of calories as a one-ounce slice of bread or one-third cup of cooked rice. Note that protein sources vary widely in calories based on their fat content, even within the very lean and lean protein categories. Very lean proteins are denoted in the menu plans as "VL protein," whereas lean proteins are called "protein"; medium-fat proteins are designated as such. In addition, the preparation of food plays a large role in its calorie content, and in the case of prepared or restaurant foods, you may not have enough information to make a completely accurate judgment about the total number of calories in a meal. Try to be careful not to underestimate the number of calories in your meals, which studies suggest is the tendency when trying to lose weight. Although we have used the 1995 American Dietetic Association Exchange List for Meal Planning as a guide for servings, in some cases our dietitians, Janet and Kathy, used their judgment and experience to make modest adjustments to the calorie levels. See Chapter 14 for more on this subject.

For the Lactose Intolerant

A significant number of Americans, especially those who are not of northern European descent, cannot eat dairy products without becoming gaseous or experiencing abdominal cramps and diarrhea. This is because their bodies do not produce the *lactase* enzyme that is necessary to break down *lactose*, one of the sugars that is present in milk.

Because calcium is an essential part of a well-balanced diet, and most people find it easiest to obtain from dairy products, the Getting Healthy menu plans contain about two milk servings per day. Many people who are lactose intolerant can still get their calcium from yogurt and certain hard cheeses because most of the lactose is predigested. If intestinal or abdominal discomfort make this impossible for you, try Lactaid milk, a commercial product that comes in regular, low-fat, and skim varieties and includes the lactase enzyme. You might also have luck with the tablet form of lactase, commercially known as Lactaid or Dairy Ease, which you chew whenever you consume dairy products.

THE BUTTER/MARGARINE DEBATE

If you are one of those people who can't tolerate a slice of plain toast, you may be confused by recent assertions that margarine is no healthier than butter. For years, the standard nutritional advice has been to avoid butter because it is high in saturated fat. Now, some scientists are saying hydrogenated margarine, which produces trans-fatty acids, also raises blood cholesterol levels. This is still controversial, but my advice is to read the label and use tub margarines made with nonhydrogenated oils. Better still, smear a bit of olive oil on your bread—this has become quite fashionable in some restaurants and you may be surprised to discover how tasty it is.

❖ MONDAY / 1,200 CALORIES ❖

MEAL	MENU	COMPOSITION	CALORIES
Breakfast	½ small banana	1 fruit	60
	1 cup bran flakes	2 starch	160
	1 cup skim milk	1 milk	90
			310
Lunch	1 serving tuna salad*	3 VL protein†	105
		1 fat	45
		1 vegetable	25
	2 slices light whole-grain bread	1 starch	80
	Fresh apple	1 fruit	60
			315
Snack	¼ cup one-percent-fat cottage cheese	½ milk	45
	4 fat-free crackers	½ starch	40
			85
Dinner	3 ounces chicken tarragon*	3 protein	165
	Medium baked potato (6 ounces)	2 starch	160
	1 cup cooked spinach	2 vegetable	50
	1 cup vegetable salad*	1 vegetable	25
	1½ tablespoons apple-cider dressing*	—	—
			400
Snack	Fresh orange	1 fruit	60
		TOTAL	**1,170**

Recipe is provided in Chapter 13.
†*VL protein = very lean protein*

For a 1,500-calorie menu, add:

Breakfast	2 slices light whole-grain toast	1 starch	80
	1 teaspoon margarine or 1 tablespoon light margarine	1 fat	45
Snack	Fresh pear	1 fruit	60
Dinner	1 ounce chicken tarragon	1 protein	55
Snack	3 cups air-popped or microwave popcorn	1 starch	80
		TOTAL	**1,490**

For an 1,800-calorie menu, add to 1,500-calorie menu:

Breakfast	½ small banana	1 fruit	60
Lunch	Add 2 ounces flaked tuna to tuna salad	2 VL protein[†]	70
	Substitute regular whole-grain bread for light	1 starch	80
Snack	2 rice cakes	1 starch	80
Dinner	1 teaspoon margarine or 1 tablespoon light margarine	1 fat	45
		TOTAL	**1,825**

[†]*VL protein = very lean protein*

❖ Tuesday / 1,200 Calories ❖

Meal	Menu	Composition	Calories
Breakfast	1 cup fresh berries	1 fruit	60
	1 English muffin	2 starch	160
	½ cup one-percent-fat cottage cheese	1 milk	90
	1 teaspoon all-fruit jelly	—	15
			325
Lunch	3 ounces broiled, skinless chicken breast	3 protein	165
	2 cups vegetable salad*	2 vegetable	50
	1½ tablespoons low-calorie vinaigrette*	1 fat	45
	1 bread stick	½ starch	40
	1 cup cubed cantaloupe	1 fruit	60
			360
Snack	1 cup skim milk	1 milk	90
Dinner	3 ounces poached salmon*	3 protein	165
		1 vegetable	25
	1 tablespoon yogurt-dill sauce*	—	5
	⅔ cup cooked brown rice	2 starch	160
	½ cup steamed broccoli	1 vegetable	25
	1 cup vegetable salad*	1 vegetable	25
	Balsamic vinegar	—	—
			405
Snack	Fresh apple	1 fruit	60
		TOTAL	**1,240**

---

*Recipe is provided in Chapter 13.

For a 1,500-calorie meal, add:

Snack	2 rice cakes	1 starch	80
Dinner	1 teaspoon margarine or 1 tablespoon light margarine	1 fat	45
	2 tangerines	1 fruit	60
Snack	3 cups air-popped or microwave popcorn	1 starch	80
		TOTAL	**1,505**

For an 1,800-calorie menu, add to 1,500-calorie menu:

Lunch	1 ounce broiled, skinless chicken breast	1 protein	55
Snack	Fresh pear	1 fruit	60
Dinner	1 ounce salmon	1 protein	55
	⅓ cup cooked brown rice	1 starch	80
		TOTAL	**1,755**

❖ WEDNESDAY / 1,200 CALORIES ❖

MEAL	MENU	COMPOSITION	CALORIES
Breakfast	1 cup shredded wheat	2 starch	160
	1 cup skim milk	1 milk	90
	Fresh orange	1 fruit	60
			310
Lunch	Low-calorie microwave		
	meal	2½ protein	140
		1 vegetable	25
		1 starch	80
	1 cup raw vegetables	1 vegetable	25
	Balsamic vinegar	—	—
	Fresh pear	1 fruit	60
			330
Snack	1½ cups chocolate shake*	1 milk	90
Dinner	1 serving chicken stir-fry*	3 protein	165
		3 vegetable	75
		1 fat	45
	⅔ cup bulgur*	2 starch	160
			445
Snack	Fresh apple	1 fruit	60
		TOTAL	*1,235*

Recipe is provided in Chapter 13.

For a 1,500-calorie menu, add:

Breakfast	2 slices light whole-grain toast	1 starch	80
	1 teaspoon margarine or 1 tablespoon light margarine	1 fat	45
Dinner	Add 1 ounce chicken breast to chicken stir-fry	1 protein	55
	⅓ cup bulgur	1 starch	80
		TOTAL	**1,495**

For an 1,800-calorie menu, add to 1,500-calorie menu:

Lunch	Small (mini) pita bread	1 starch	80
Snack	1 cup berries	1 fruit	60
Dinner	Add 1 ounce chicken breast to chicken stir-fry	1 protein	55
	1 cup cubed cantaloupe	1 fruit	60
		TOTAL	**1,750**

❖ THURSDAY / 1,200 CALORIES ❖

MEAL	MENU	COMPOSITION	CALORIES
Breakfast	½ cup fresh fruit salad	1 fruit	60
	1 cup oatmeal	2 starch	160
	1 cup skim milk	1 milk	90
			310
Lunch	4 ounces smoked skinless turkey breast	4 VL protein†	140
	2 slices whole-grain bread	2 starch	160
	1 teaspoon mustard	—	—
	Lettuce and tomato slices	1 vegetable	25
	1½ tablespoons Dijon dressing*	1 fat	45
	2 tangerines	1 fruit	60
			430
Snack	1 cup plain or artificially sweetened nonfat yogurt	1 milk	90
Dinner	1 cup cooked pasta	2 starch	160
	½ cup meat sauce*	1 protein	55
		1½ vegetable	40
	2 cups vegetable salad*	2 vegetable	50
	1½ tablespoons low-calorie vinaigrette*	1 fat	45
			350
Snack	Fresh pear	1 fruit	60
		TOTAL	**1,240**

---

*Recipe is provided in Chapter 13.
†VL protein = very lean protein

For a 1,500-calorie menu, add:

Snack	Fresh apple	1 fruit	60
Dinner	1 cup cooked pasta	2 starch	160
	½ cup meat sauce	1 protein	55
		1½ vegetable	40
		TOTAL	**1,555**

For an 1,800-calorie menu, add to 1,500-calorie menu:

Breakfast	½ cup fresh fruit salad	1 fruit	60
Lunch	1 ounce turkey breast	1 VL protein†	35
Dinner	½ cup asparagus	1 vegetable	25
	10 stuffed green olives	1 fat	45
Snack	¾ ounce pretzels	1 starch	80
		TOTAL	**1,800**

---

†*VL protein = very lean protein*

◆ FRIDAY / 1,200 CALORIES ◆

MEAL	MENU	COMPOSITION	CALORIES
Breakfast	½ medium grapefruit	1 fruit	60
	1 cup Cream of Wheat	2 starch	160
	1 cup skim milk	1 milk	90
			310
Lunch	1 serving chef's salad*	2 VL protein†	70
		1 protein	55
		3 vegetable	75
	1½ tablespoons low-calorie vinaigrette*	1 fat	45
	4 melba toast	1 starch	80
	Fresh apple	1 fruit	60
			385
Snack	1 cup reduced-fat hot cocoa	½ milk	45
	1½ cups air-popped or microwave popcorn	½ starch	40
			85
Dinner	4 ounces tangy flounder*	4 VL protein†	140
	1 cup cooked peas	2 starch	160
	1 cup vegetable salad*	1 vegetable	25
	1½ tablespoons apple-cider dressing*	—	—
	½ cup cooked cauliflower	1 vegetable	25
			350
Snack	2 tangerines	1 fruit	60
		TOTAL	**1,190**

---

*Recipe is provided in Chapter 13.
†VL protein = very lean protein

For a 1,500-calorie menu, add:

Breakfast	2 slices light whole-grain toast	1 starch	80
	1 teaspoon margarine or 1 tablespoon light margarine	1 fat	45
Lunch	4 melba toast	1 starch	80
Snack	Fresh pear	1 fruit	60
		TOTAL	**1,455**

For an 1,800-calorie menu, add to 1,500-calorie menu:

Breakfast	½ medium grapefruit	1 fruit	60
Snack	3 cups air-popped or microwave popcorn	1 starch	80
Dinner	3 ounces tangy flounder	3 VL protein†	105
	1 teaspoon olive oil	1 fat	45
		TOTAL	**1,745**

---

†*VL protein = very lean protein*

❖ SATURDAY / 1,200 CALORIES ❖

MEAL	MENU	COMPOSITION	CALORIES
Breakfast	1 cup raisin bran	2 starch	160
		½ fruit	30
	1 cup skim milk	1 milk	90
			280
Lunch	3 ounces lean ground beef	3 protein	165
	Hamburger roll	2 starch	160
	Lettuce and tomato slices	1 vegetable	25
	Fresh apple	1 fruit	60
			410
Snack	1 cup raw vegetables	1 vegetable	25
	4 fat-free crackers	½ starch	40
	¼ cup spinach-yogurt dip*	¼ milk +	
		½ vegetable	35
			100
Dinner	4 ounces skinless turkey breast	4 VL protein†	140
	1 serving cottage fries*	1 starch	80
	1 cup green beans	2 vegetable	50
	2 cups vegetable salad*	2 vegetable	50
	1½ tablespoons low-calorie vinaigrette dressing*	1 fat	45
			365
Snack	Fresh orange	1 fruit	60
		TOTAL	**1,215**

---

*Recipe is provided in Chapter 13.
†VL protein = very lean protein

For a 1,500-calorie menu, add:

Breakfast	2 slices light whole-grain toast	1 starch	80
	1 teaspoon margarine or 1 tablespoon light margarine	1 fat	45
Snack	Fresh peach	1 fruit	60
Dinner	1 ounce skinless turkey breast	1 VL protein†	35
	1 serving cottage fries	1 starch	80
		TOTAL	**1,515**

For an 1,800-calorie menu, add to 1,500-calorie menu:

Lunch	1 ounce ground beef	1 protein	55
Snack	4 fat-free crackers	½ starch	40
Dinner	1 serving cottage fries	1 starch	80
	1 teaspoon olive oil	1 fat	45
	Fresh pear	1 fruit	60
		TOTAL	**1,795**

---

†*VL protein = very lean protein*

◆ Sunday / 1,200 Calories ◆

Meal	Menu	Composition	Calories
Breakfast	Fresh orange	1 fruit	60
	½ cup cooked cereal	1 starch	80
	2 slices light whole-grain toast	1 starch	80
	1 teaspoon margarine or 1 tablespoon light margarine	1 fat	45
	1 poached egg	1 medium-fat protein	75
			340
Lunch	½ cup one-percent-fat cottage cheese	1 milk	90
	½ cup fresh fruit salad	1 fruit	60
	2 cups vegetable salad*	2 vegetable	50
	2 tablespoons fat-free salad dressing	—	25
	Small (mini) pita bread	1 starch	80
			305
Snack	Fresh pear	1 fruit	60
Dinner	4 ounces grilled shrimp	4 VL protein†	140
	1 ear fresh corn (large)	2 starch	160
	1 cup steamed broccoli	2 vegetable	50
	1 teaspoon olive oil	1 fat	45
			395
Snack	1 cup skim milk	1 milk	90
		TOTAL	**1,190**

Recipe is provided in Chapter 13.
†*VL protein = very lean protein*

For a 1,500-calorie menu, add:

Lunch	¼ cup one-percent-fat cottage cheese	½ milk	45
	½ cup fresh fruit salad	1 fruit	60
Snack	2 rice cakes	1 starch	80
Dinner	1 teaspoon olive oil	1 fat	45
Snack	¾ cup corn flakes	1 starch	80
		TOTAL	**1,500**

For an 1,800-calorie menu, add to 1,500-calorie menu:

Lunch	Substitute large pita bread for small	1 starch	80
	1 teaspoon margarine or 1 tablespoon light margarine	1 fat	45
Dinner	2 ounces grilled shrimp	2 VL protein†	70
	Fresh apple	1 fruit	60
Snack	1 cup cubed honeydew melon	1 fruit	60
		TOTAL	**1,815**

---

†*VL protein = very lean protein*

❖ MONDAY / 1,200 CALORIES ❖

MEAL	MENU	COMPOSITION	CALORIES
Breakfast	½ medium grapefruit	1 fruit	60
	1 cup shredded wheat	2 starch	160
	1 cup skim milk	1 milk	90
			310
Lunch	1½ cups canned, low-fat lentil soup	1½ VL protein†	55
		1½ starch	120
	Small whole-grain pita	1 starch	80
	1 cup raw vegetables	1 vegetable	25
	¼ cup spinach-yogurt dip*	¼ milk + ½ vegetable	35
			315
Snack	¼ cup one-percent-fat cottage cheese	½ milk	45
	8 fat-free crackers	1 starch	80
			125
Dinner	5 ounces broiled sole	5 VL protein†	175
	1 tablespoon lemon-yogurt dressing*	—	10
	⅓ cup bulgur*	1 starch	80
	1 teaspoon olive oil	1 fat	45
	2 cups vegetable salad*	2 vegetable	50
	1½ tablespoons apple-cider dressing*	—	—
	½ cup cooked zucchini	1 vegetable	25
			385
Snack	Fresh pear	1 fruit	60
		TOTAL	**1,195**

---

*Recipe is provided in Chapter 13.
†VL protein = very lean protein

For a 1,500-calorie menu, add:

Breakfast	1 slice whole-grain toast	1 starch	80
	1 teaspoon margarine or 1 tablespoon light margarine	1 fat	45
Snack	2 tangerines	1 fruit	60
Dinner	⅓ cup bulgur	1 starch	80
	½ cup cooked zucchini	1 vegetable	25
		TOTAL	**1,485**

For an 1,800-calorie menu, add to 1,500-calorie menu:

Dinner	3 ounces broiled sole	3 VL protein†	105
	⅓ cup bulgur	1 starch	80
	1 teaspoon olive oil	1 fat	45
	1 cup berries	1 fruit	60
		TOTAL	**1,775**

---

†*VL protein = very lean protein*

❖ TUESDAY / 1,200 CALORIES ❖

MEAL	MENU	COMPOSITION	CALORIES
Breakfast	1 cup fresh berries	1 fruit	60
	1 cup plain or artificially sweetened nonfat yogurt	1 milk	90
	1 slice whole-grain toast	1 starch	80
	1 teaspoon all-fruit jelly	—	15
			245
Lunch	1 serving tuna salad*	3 VL protein†	105
		1 fat	45
		1 vegetable	25
	2 slices whole-grain bread	2 starch	160
	Fresh apple	1 fruit	60
			395
Snack	½ cup skim milk	½ milk	45
	2 popcorn-flavored rice cakes	1 starch	80
			125
Dinner	3 ounces honey-mustard chicken*	3 protein	165
	1 cup vegetable rice pilaf*	2 vegetable	50
		1 starch	80
	2 cups vegetable salad*	2 vegetable	50
	Balsamic vinegar	—	—
			345
Snack	Fresh orange	1 fruit	60
		TOTAL	**1,170**

---

*Recipe is provided in Chapter 13.
†VL protein = very lean protein

For a 1,500-calorie menu, add:

Breakfast	1 slice whole-grain toast	1 starch	80
Snack	Fresh pear	1 fruit	60
Dinner	Add 1 ounce skinless chicken breast to honey-mustard chicken	1 protein	55
	1 teaspoon olive oil	1 fat	45
Snack	3 cups air-popped or microwave popcorn	1 starch	80
		TOTAL	**1,490**

For an 1,800-calorie menu, add to 1,500-calorie menu:

Lunch	Add 1 ounce flaked tuna to tuna salad	1 VL protein†	35
Snack	1 rice cake	½ starch	40
Dinner	Add 1 ounce skinless chicken breast to honey-mustard chicken	1 protein	55
	1 cup vegetable rice pilaf	1 starch	80
		2 vegetable	50
	½ medium grapefruit	1 fruit	60
		TOTAL	**1,810**

---

†*VL protein = very lean protein*

❖ WEDNESDAY / 1,200 CALORIES ❖

MEAL	MENU	COMPOSITION	CALORIES
Breakfast	½ medium grapefruit	1 fruit	60
	1 cup bran flakes	2 starch	160
	1 cup skim milk	1 milk	90
			310
Lunch	1 serving zesty chicken salad*	3 protein	165
		1 vegetable	25
	Large whole-wheat pita	2 starch	160
	1 large lettuce leaf and 1 medium tomato	1 vegetable	25
	Fresh apple	1 fruit	60
			435
Snack	1½ cups chocolate shake*	1 milk	90
Dinner	3 ounces tangy sole*	3 VL protein†	105
	1 serving cottage fries*	1 starch	80
	1 teaspoon margarine or 1 tablespoon light margarine	1 fat	45
	½ cup steamed spinach	1 vegetable	25
	2 cups vegetable salad*	2 vegetable	50
	Balsamic vinegar	—	—
			305
Snack	Fresh orange	1 fruit	60
		TOTAL	1,200

---

*Recipe is provided in Chapter 13.
†VL protein = very lean protein

For a 1,500-calorie menu, add:

Dinner	2 ounces tangy sole	2 VL protein[†]	70
	1 serving of cottage fries	1 starch	80
	1 teaspoon olive oil	1 fat	45
	Fresh apple	1 fruit	60
		TOTAL	**1,455**

For an 1,800-calorie menu, add to 1,500-calorie menu:

Breakfast	½ medium grapefruit	1 fruit	60
Lunch	Add 1 ounce chicken breast to zesty chicken salad	1 protein	55
Dinner	1 serving cottage fries	1 starch	80
	1 ½ tablespoons low-calorie vinaigrette*	1 fat	45
Snack	2 rice cakes	1 starch	80
		TOTAL	**1,775**

---

*Recipe is provided in Chapter 13.
[†]VL protein = very lean protein

❖ THURSDAY / 1,200 CALORIES ❖

MEAL	MENU	COMPOSITION	CALORIES
Breakfast	½ small banana	1 fruit	60
	1 cup cooked oatmeal	2 starch	160
	1 cup skim milk	1 milk	90
			310
Lunch	1 serving chef's salad*	2 VL protein†	70
		1 protein	55
		3 vegetable	75
	1½ tablespoons low-calorie vinaigrette*	1 fat	45
	Fresh apple	1 fruit	60
			305
Snack	Fresh pear	1 fruit	60
Dinner	1½ cups cooked pasta	3 starch	240
	1 cup eggplant sauce*	½ protein	30
		3 vegetable	75
		½ fat	20
	1 cup vegetable salad*	1 vegetable	25
	2 tablespoons fat-free salad dressing	—	25
			415
Snack	1 slice light whole-grain bread	½ starch	40
	1 slice fat-free cheese	½ milk	45
			85
		TOTAL	1,175

---

*Recipe is provided in Chapter 13.
†VL protein = very lean protein

For a 1,500-calorie menu, add:

Breakfast	1 teaspoon margarine or 1 tablespoon light margarine	1 fat	45
Lunch	Add 1 ounce turkey to chef's salad	1 VL protein†	35
	2 bread sticks	1 starch	80
Dinner	½ cup cooked pasta	1 starch	80
	Fresh orange	1 fruit	60
		TOTAL	**1,475**

For an 1,800-calorie menu, add to 1,500-calorie menu:

Breakfast	½ small banana	1 fruit	60
Lunch	Add 1 ounce lean roast beef to chef's salad	1 protein	55
Dinner	½ cup cooked pasta	1 starch	80
	½ cup eggplant sauce	¼ protein	15
		1½ vegetable	40
		¼ fat	10
	1 teaspoon olive oil	1 fat	45
		TOTAL	**1,780**

---

†VL protein = very lean protein

❖ FRIDAY / 1,200 CALORIES ❖

MEAL	MENU	COMPOSITION	CALORIES
Breakfast	Fresh orange	1 fruit	60
	2 slices whole-grain toast	2 starch	160
	1 teaspoon all-fruit jelly	—	15
	½ cup one-percent-fat		
	cottage cheese	1 milk	90
			325
Lunch	Low-calorie microwave meal	2½ protein	140
		2 vegetable	50
		1 starch	80
	2 cups vegetable salad*	2 vegetable	50
	1½ tablespoons apple-cider		
	dressing*	—	—
			320
Snack	½ cup skim milk	½ milk	45
	1½ cups air-popped		
	or microwave popcorn	½ starch	40
			85
Dinner	3 ounces lean steak	3 protein	165
	2 servings cottage fries*	2 starch	160
	1 cup vegetable salad*	1 vegetable	25
	1½ tablespoons low-calorie		
	vinaigrette dressing*	1 fat	45
	Fresh apple	1 fruit	60
			455
Snack	Fresh pear	1 fruit	60
		TOTAL	**1,245**

---

*Recipe is provided in Chapter 13.

For a 1,500-calorie menu, add:

Lunch	Small (mini) pita bread	1 starch	80
	1 teaspoon margarine or 1 tablespoon light margarine	1 fat	45
Snack	1 cup fresh strawberries	1 fruit	60
Snack	2 rice cakes	1 starch	80
		TOTAL	**1,510**

For an 1,800-calorie menu, add to 1,500-calorie menu:

Breakfast	1 teaspoon margarine or 1 tablespoon light margarine	1 fat	45
Lunch	½ medium grapefruit	1 fruit	60
Dinner	2 ounces lean steak	2 protein	110
	1 serving cottage fries	1 starch	80
		TOTAL	**1,805**

❖ SUNDAY / 1,200 CALORIES ❖

MEAL	MENU	COMPOSITION	CALORIES
Breakfast	½ medium grapefruit	1 fruit	60
	2-egg-white omelette	1 VL protein†	35
	½ cup cooked peppers/onions	1 vegetable	25
	2 slices light whole-grain toast	1 starch	80
	1 teaspoon margarine or 1 tablespoon light margarine	1 fat	45
	1 teaspoon all-fruit jelly	—	15
			260
Lunch	2 ounces water-packed flaked salmon	2 protein	110
	2 cups vegetable salad*	2 vegetable	50
	1½ teaspoons Dijon dressing*	1 fat	45
	Small (mini) pita bread	1 starch	80
	Fresh pear	1 fruit	60
			345
Snack	Fresh apple	1 fruit	60
Dinner	1 cup turkey chili*	3 protein	165
		1 vegetable	25
		2 starch	160
	⅓ cup cooked brown rice	1 starch	80
	1 cup vegetable salad*	1 vegetable	25
	Balsamic vinegar	—	—
			455
Snack	1 cup skim milk	1 milk	90
		TOTAL	**1,210**

---

*Recipe is provided in Chapter 13.

†VL protein = very lean protein

For a 1,500-calorie menu, add:

Snack	2 rice cakes	1 starch	80
Dinner	1 ounce ground turkey burger	1 protein	55
	1 teaspoon olive oil	1 fat	45
	1 cup fresh berries	1 fruit	60
Snack	3 cups air-popped or microwave popcorn	1 starch	80
		TOTAL	**1,520**

For an 1,800-calorie menu, add to 1,500-calorie menu:

Breakfast	1 teaspoon margarine or 1 tablespoon light margarine	1 fat	45
Lunch	Add 1 ounce flaked tuna to tuna salad	1 VL protein†	35
	Substitute regular whole-grain toast for light toast	1 starch	80
Snack	½ medium grapefruit	1 fruit	60
Dinner	1 ounce ground turkey burger	1 protein	55
		TOTAL	**1,795**

---

†VL protein = very lean protein

❖ SATURDAY / 1,200 CALORIES ❖

MEAL	MENU	COMPOSITION	CALORIES
Breakfast	Fresh orange	1 fruit	60
	1 English muffin	2 starch	160
	1 teaspoon all-fruit jelly	—	15
	½ cup one-percent-fat cottage cheese	1 milk	90
			325
Lunch	1 serving tuna salad*	3 VL protein†	105
		1 fat	45
		1 vegetable	25
	2 slices light whole-grain toast	1 starch	80
	Fresh apple	1 fruit	60
			315
Snack	1 cup raw vegetables	1 vegetable	25
	¼ cup spinach-yogurt dip*	¼ milk + ½ vegetable	35
	4 fat-free crackers	½ starch	40
			100
Dinner	3 ounces ground turkey burger	3 protein	165
	Hamburger roll	2 starch	160
	2 cups vegetable salad*	2 vegetable	50
	Balsamic vinegar	—	—
	½ cup steamed broccoli	1 vegetable	25
			400
Snack	Fresh pear	1 fruit	60
		TOTAL	**1,200**

---

*Recipe is provided in Chapter 13.
†VL protein = very lean protein

For a 1,500-calorie menu, add:

Breakfast	½ medium grapefruit	1 fruit	60
Lunch	1 ounce flaked salmon	1 protein	55
	1 teaspoon olive oil	1 fat	45
Snack	2 rice cakes	1 starch	80
Dinner	⅓ cup cooked brown rice	1 starch	80
		TOTAL	**1,530**

For an 1,800-calorie menu, add to 1,500-calorie menu:

Dinner	½ cup chili	1½ protein	85
		½ vegetable	15
		1 starch	80
	1 teaspoon olive oil	1 fat	45
Snack	1 cup fresh strawberries	1 fruit	60
		TOTAL	**1,815**

12

MENU PLAN II: THE LOWER GLYCEMIC INDEX APPROACH

❖

If you have not achieved a weight loss of at least 4 pounds after two months on Menu Plan I, make sure that you calculated the calories you need properly. If you did, and you have conformed honestly to the menu plan, you may want to switch to Menu Plan II, the lower glycemic index approach. Here you'll find balanced meals that emphasize fibrous vegetables and legumes, rather than simple carbohydrates and starches such as products made from refined flours and white potatoes. Menu Plan II also has a slightly higher protein and fat content.

This is the approximate composition of the Getting Healthy lower glycemic index diet:

1,200 calories
  6 servings of protein
  3 servings of starch
  2 servings of milk
10 servings of vegetables
  2 servings of fruit
  2 servings of fat

In the 1,200-calorie lower glycemic index diet, 21 percent of your calories come from fat, 30 percent from protein, and 49 percent from carbohydrates.

1,500 calories
  8 servings of protein
  4 servings of starch
  2 servings of milk
10 servings of vegetables
  3 servings of fruit
  4 servings of fat

In the 1,500-calorie lower glycemic index diet, approximately 27 percent of your calories come from fat, 25 percent from protein, and 48 percent from carbohydrates.

1,800 calories
  9 servings of protein
  5 servings of starch
  2 servings of milk
10 servings of vegetables
  4 servings of fruit
  5 servings of fat

In the 1,800-calorie lower glycemic index diet, approximately 26 percent of your calories come from fat, 26 percent from protein, and 48 percent from carbohydrates.

❖ MONDAY / 1,200 CALORIES ❖

MEAL	MENU	COMPOSITION	CALORIES
Breakfast	1 cup tomato juice	2 vegetable	50
	½ cup All-Bran cereal	1 starch	80
	1 cup skim milk	1 milk	90
			220
Lunch	1 serving tuna salad*	3 VL protein†	105
		1 fat	45
		1 vegetable	25
	2 cups vegetable salad*	2 vegetable	50
	Balsamic vinegar	—	—
	Fresh pear	1 fruit	60
			285
Snack	½ cup one-percent-fat cottage cheese	1 milk	90
	4 whole-grain fat-free crackers	½ starch	40
			130
Dinner	3 ounces chicken tarragon*	3 protein	165
	⅔ cup cooked black beans	2 starch	160
	1 cup cooked spinach	2 vegetable	50
	1 teaspoon margarine or 1 tablespoon light margarine	1 fat	45
	3 cups vegetable salad*	3 vegetable	75
	1½ tablespoons apple-cider dressing*	—	—
			495
Snack	Fresh orange	1 fruit	60
		TOTAL	**1,190**

*Recipe is provided in Chapter 13.
†VL protein = very lean protein

For a 1,500-calorie menu, add:

Lunch	1 slice pumpernickel bread	1 starch	80
	1 teaspoon margarine or 1 tablespoon light margarine	1 fat	45
Snack	1 cup strawberries	1 fruit	60
Dinner	Add 2 ounces skinless, boneless chicken to chicken tarragon	2 protein	110
	1 teaspoon olive oil	1 fat	45
		TOTAL	**1,530**

For an 1,800-calorie menu, add to 1,500-calorie menu:

Breakfast	½ cup All-Bran cereal	1 starch	80
Lunch	Add 2 ounces flaked tuna to tuna salad	2 VL protein†	70
Dinner	10 green stuffed olives	1 fat	45
	Fresh apple	1 fruit	60
		TOTAL	**1,785**

---

†*VL protein = very lean protein*

◆ TUESDAY / 1,200 CALORIES ◆

MEAL	MENU	COMPOSITION	CALORIES
Breakfast	1 cup vegetable juice	2 vegetable	50
	2 slices light whole-grain toast	1 starch	80
	½ cup one-percent-fat cottage cheese	1 milk	90
			220
Lunch	3 ounces grilled, skinless chicken breast	3 protein	165
	3 cups vegetable salad*	3 vegetable	75
	1½ tablespoons low-calorie vinaigrette*	1 fat	45
	Fresh apple	1 fruit	60
			345
Snack	1 cup skim milk	1 milk	90
Dinner	3 ounces poached salmon*	3 protein	165
		1 vegetable	25
	1 tablespoon yogurt-dill sauce*	—	5
	⅔ cup cooked brown rice	2 starch	160
	1 teaspoon margarine or 1 tablespoon light margarine	1 fat	45
	2 cups vegetable salad*	2 vegetable	50
	2 tablespoons fat-free salad dressing	—	25
	1 cup steamed broccoli with lemon	2 vegetable	50
			525
Snack	1 cup cubed cantaloupe	1 fruit	60
		TOTAL	**1,240**

*Recipe is provided in Chapter 13.

For a 1,500-calorie menu, add:

Breakfast	1 teaspoon margarine or 1 tablespoon light margarine	1 fat	45
Lunch	2 bread sticks	1 starch	80
Dinner	2 ounces poached salmon	2 protein	110
	1 teaspoon olive oil	1 fat	45
		TOTAL	**1,520**

For an 1,800-calorie menu, add to 1,500-calorie menu:

Breakfast	½ medium grapefruit	1 fruit	60
	½ cup oatmeal	1 starch	80
Lunch	1 ounce grilled, skinless chicken breast	1 protein	55
Dinner	1 teaspoon olive oil	1 fat	45
	Fresh orange	1 fruit	60
		TOTAL	**1,820**

✦ WEDNESDAY / 1,200 CALORIES ✦

MEAL	MENU	COMPOSITION	CALORIES
Breakfast	1 cup plain or artificially sweetened nonfat yogurt	1 milk	90
	1 cup berries	1 fruit	60
			150
Lunch	Low-calorie microwave meal	2½ protein	140
		2 vegetable	50
		1 starch	80
	2 cups vegetable salad*	2 vegetable	50
	1½ tablespoons low-calorie vinaigrette*	1 fat	45
			365
Snack	1½ cups chocolate shake*	1 milk	90
Dinner	1 serving chicken stir-fry*	3 protein	165
		3 vegetable	75
		1 fat	45
	⅔ cup cooked brown rice	2 starch	160
			445
Snack	1 cup fresh strawberries	1 fruit	60
	2 slices fat-free cheese	1 milk	90
			150
		TOTAL	**1,200**

---

*Recipe is provided in Chapter 13.

For a 1,500-calorie menu, add:

Breakfast	2 slices light whole-grain toast	1 starch	80
	1 teaspoon margarine or 1 tablespoon light margarine	1 fat	45
Lunch	Fresh apple	1 fruit	60
Dinner	2 ounces chicken breast	2 protein	110
		TOTAL	**1,495**

For an 1,800-calorie menu, add to 1,500-calorie menu:

Breakfast	1 scrambled egg	1 medium-fat protein	75
	1 teaspoon margarine or 1 tablespoon light margarine	1 fat	45
Dinner	⅓ cup cooked brown rice	1 starch	80
	2 tangerines	1 fruit	60
		TOTAL	**1,755**

❖ Thursday / 1,200 Calories ❖

MEAL	MENU	COMPOSITION	CALORIES
Breakfast	½ cup oatmeal	1 starch	80
	1 teaspoon margarine or 1 tablespoon light margarine	1 fat	45
	1 cup skim milk	1 milk	90
			215
Lunch	3 ounces smoked skinless turkey breast	3 VL protein†	105
	2 slices light whole-grain bread	1 starch	80
	1 teaspoon mustard	—	—
	2 cups lettuce and tomato slices	2 vegetable	50
	2 tablespoons fat-free dressing	—	25
			260
Snack	1 cup raw vegetables	1 vegetable	25
	½ cup spinach-yogurt dip*	½ milk + 1 vegetable	70
	4 whole-grain fat-free crackers	½ starch	40
			135
Dinner	3 ounces lean beef	3 protein	165
	½ cup corn	1 starch	80
	3 cups vegetable salad*	3 vegetable	75
	1 cup asparagus	2 vegetable	50
	1 teaspoon olive oil	1 fat	45
	Fresh apple	1 fruit	60
			475
Snack	½ medium grapefruit	1 fruit	60
	¼ cup one-percent-fat cottage cheese	½ milk	45
			105
		TOTAL	**1,190**

---

*Recipe is provided in Chapter 13.
†VL protein = very lean protein

For a 1,500-calorie menu, add:

Breakfast	1 cup vegetable juice	2 vegetable	50
Lunch	Fresh peach	1 fruit	60
Dinner	2 ounces lean beef	2 protein	110
	½ cup corn	1 starch	80
		TOTAL	**1,490**

For an 1,800-calorie menu, add to 1,500-calorie menu:

Breakfast	1 cup cubed cantaloupe	1 fruit	60
Lunch	2 ounces turkey breast	2 VL protein†	70
	½ cup sweet potato	1 starch	80
	1 teaspoon margarine or 1 tablespoon light margarine	1 fat	45
Dinner	10 stuffed green olives	1 fat	45
		TOTAL	**1,790**

---

†*VL protein = very lean protein*

❖ FRIDAY / 1,200 CALORIES ❖

MEAL	MENU	COMPOSITION	CALORIES
Breakfast	1 cup vegetable juice	2 vegetable	50
	½ cup Cream of Wheat	1 starch	80
	1 cup skim milk	1 milk	90
			220
Lunch	1 serving chef's salad*	2 VL protein†	70
		1 protein	55
		3 vegetable	75
	1½ tablespoons low-calorie vinaigrette*	1 fat	45
	4 melba toast	1 starch	80
			325
Snack	1 slice light whole-grain toast	½ starch	40
	2 slices fat-free cheese	1 milk	90
			130
Dinner	4 ounces tangy flounder*	4 VL protein†	140
	½ cup cooked peas	1 starch	80
	1 cup cooked cauliflower	2 vegetable	50
	2 cups vegetable salad*	2 vegetable	50
	1½ tablespoons low-calorie vinaigrette	1 fat	45
	Fresh orange	1 fruit	60
			425
Snack	½ grapefruit	1 fruit	60
		TOTAL	**1,160**

---

*Recipe is provided in Chapter 13.
†VL protein = very lean protein

For a 1,500-calorie menu, add:

Breakfast	1 teaspoon margarine or 1 tablespoon light margarine	1 fat	45
Snack	1 cup cubed cantaloupe	1 fruit	60
Dinner	2 ounces tangy flounder	2 VL protein[†]	70
	½ cup cooked peas	1 starch	80
	1 teaspoon margarine	1 fat	45
		TOTAL	**1,460**

For an 1,800-calorie menu, add to 1,500-calorie menu:

Breakfast	½ cup Cream of Wheat	1 starch	80
Lunch	Add 1 ounce lean roast beef to chef's salad	1 protein	55
	1 teaspoon olive oil	1 fat	45
Snack	Fresh apple	1 fruit	60
	1 cup plain or artificially sweetened nonfat yogurt	1 milk	90
		TOTAL	**1,790**

[†]*VL protein = very lean protein*

❖ SATURDAY / 1,200 CALORIES ❖

MEAL	MENU	COMPOSITION	CALORIES
Breakfast	2-egg-white omelette	1 VL protein†	35
	½ cup cooked mushrooms/ onions	1 vegetable	25
	2 slices light whole-grain toast	1 starch	80
	1 teaspoon margarine or 1 tablespoon light margarine	1 fat	45
			185
Lunch	3 ounces lean ground beef	3 protein	165
	1 slice pumpernickel bread	1 starch	80
	1 cup lettuce and tomato slices	1 vegetable	25
	Fresh apple	1 fruit	60
			330
Snack	1 cup raw vegetables	1 vegetable	25
	4 whole-grain fat-free crackers	½ starch	40
	¼ cup spinach-yogurt dip*	¼ milk + ½ vegetable	35
			100
Dinner	4 ounces skinless turkey breast	4 VL protein†	140
	½ cup sweet potato	1 starch	80
	1 cup green beans	2 vegetable	50
	3 cups vegetable salad*	3 vegetable	75
	1 teaspoon olive oil	1 fat	45
	Unlimited vinegar	—	—
	2 tangerines	1 fruit	60
			450
Snack	1 cup plain or artificially sweetened nonfat yogurt	1 milk	90
		TOTAL	**1,155**

*Recipe is provided in Chapter 13.
†VL protein = very lean protein

For a 1,500-calorie menu, add:

Lunch	1 slice pumpernickel bread	1 starch	80
Dinner	3 ounces skinless turkey breast	3 VL protein†	105
	1 teaspoon olive oil	1 fat	45
Snack	Fresh orange	1 fruit	60
		TOTAL	**1,480**

For an 1,800-calorie menu, add to 1,500-calorie menu:

Breakfast	1 whole egg	1 medium-fat protein	75
	½ medium grapefruit	1 fruit	60
Lunch	1½ tablespoons low-calorie vinaigrette*	1 fat	45
Dinner	½ cup sweet potato	1 starch	80
Snack	1 rice cake	½ starch	40
		TOTAL	**1,780**

---

*Recipe is provided in Chapter 13.
†VL protein = very lean protein

❖ Sunday / 1,200 Calories ❖

Meal	Menu	Composition	Calories
Breakfast	1 cup V-8 juice	2 vegetable	50
	1 poached egg	1 medium-fat protein	75
	2 slices light whole-grain toast	1 starch	80
	1 teaspoon margarine or 1 tablespoon light margarine	1 fat	45
			250
Lunch	½ cup one-percent-fat cottage cheese	1 milk	90
	½ cup fresh fruit salad	1 fruit	60
	2 cups vegetable salad*	2 vegetable	50
	Balsamic vinegar	—	—
	Small (mini) whole-wheat pita	1 starch	80
			280
Snack	1 cup frozen yogurt*	1 milk	90
		½ fruit	30
			120
Dinner	5 ounces grilled shrimp	5 VL protein†	175
	½ cup corn	1 starch	80
	1 teaspoon margarine or 1 tablespoon light margarine	1 fat	45
	1 cup steamed broccoli	2 vegetable	50
	2 cups vegetable salad*	2 vegetable	50
	Balsamic vinegar	—	—
	1 cup cubed honeydew melon	1 fruit	60
			460
Snack	1½ cups chocolate shake*	1 milk	90
		TOTAL	**1,200**

*Recipe is provided in Chapter 13.
†VL protein = very lean protein

For a 1,500-calorie menu, add:

Lunch	½ cup one-percent-fat cottage cheese	1 milk	90
	½ cup fresh fruit salad	1 fruit	60
Dinner	½ cup corn	1 starch	80
	1 teaspoon olive oil	1 fat	45
		TOTAL	**1,475**

For an 1,800-calorie menu, add to 1,500-calorie menu:

Breakfast	1 cup berries	1 fruit	60
Lunch	1 cup vegetable salad	1 vegetable	25
	1 teaspoon olive oil	1 fat	45
Dinner	2 ounces grilled shrimp	2 VL protein†	70
Snack	3 cups air-popped or microwave popcorn	1 starch	80
		TOTAL	**1,755**

---

†VL protein = *very lean protein*

❖ MONDAY / 1,200 CALORIES ❖

MEAL	MENU	COMPOSITION	CALORIES
Breakfast	1 cup tomato juice	2 vegetable	50
	½ cup All-Bran cereal	1 starch	80
	1 cup skim milk	1 milk	90
			220
Lunch	1 cup canned, low-fat lentil soup	1 VL protein†	35
		1 starch	80
	3 ounces grilled turkey burger	3 protein	165
	2 cups vegetable salad*	2 vegetable	50
	1½ tablespoons Dijon dressing*	1 fat	45
	Fresh apple	1 fruit	60
			435
Snack	1 cup plain or artificially sweetened nonfat yogurt	1 milk	90
Dinner	4 ounces broiled sole	4 VL protein†	140
	1 tablespoon lemon-yogurt dressing*	—	10
	⅓ cup bulgur*	1 starch	80
	1 teaspoon margarine or 1 tablespoon light margarine	1 fat	45
	2 cups vegetable salad*	2 vegetable	50
	1½ tablespoons Dijon dressing*	1 fat	45
	1 cup cooked zucchini	2 vegetable	50
			420
Snack	1 cup fresh strawberries	1 fruit	60
		TOTAL	**1,225**

---

*Recipe is provided in Chapter 13.

†VL protein = very lean protein

For a 1,500-calorie menu, add:

Snack	Fresh orange	1 fruit	60
Dinner	3 ounces broiled sole	3 VL protein[†]	105
	⅓ cup bulgur	1 starch	80
	1 teaspoon margarine or 1 tablespoon light margarine	1 fat	45
		TOTAL	**1,515**

For an 1,800-calorie menu, add to 1,500-calorie menu:

Breakfast	½ cup All-Bran cereal	1 starch	80
	½ medium grapefruit	1 fruit	60
Lunch	1 ounce grilled turkey burger	1 protein	55
Dinner	1 cup vegetable salad	1 vegetable	25
	1½ tablespoons Dijon dressing	1 fat	45
		TOTAL	**1,780**

[†] *VL protein = very lean protein*

◆ TUESDAY / 1,200 CALORIES ◆

MEAL	MENU	COMPOSITION	CALORIES
Breakfast	1 cup plain or artificially sweetened nonfat yogurt	1 milk	90
	1 cup berries	1 fruit	60
	2 slices light whole-grain toast	1 starch	80
			230
Lunch	1 serving tuna salad*	3 VL protein†	105
		1 fat	45
		1 vegetable	25
	2 slices light whole-grain bread	1 starch	80
			255
Snack	½ cup one-percent-fat cottage cheese	1 milk	90
	Fresh apple	1 fruit	60
	1 cup raw vegetables	1 vegetable	25
			175
Dinner	3 ounces chicken Dijon*	3 protein	165
	1 cup asparagus	2 vegetable	50
	1 cup vegetable rice pilaf*	1 starch	80
		2 vegetable	50
	2 cups tossed salad	2 vegetable	50
	1½ tablespoons low-calorie vinaigrette*	1 fat	45
			440
Snack	1 cup plain or artificially sweetened nonfat yogurt	1 milk	90
		TOTAL	**1,190**

---

*Recipe is provided in Chapter 13.
†VL protein = very lean protein

For a 1,500-calorie menu, add:

Dinner	2 ounces chicken Dijon	2 protein	110
	½ cup vegetable		
	rice pilaf	½ starch	40
		1 vegetable	25
	1 teaspoon olive oil	1 fat	45
Snack	2 tangerines	1 fruit	60
		TOTAL	**1,470**

For an 1,800-calorie menu, add to 1,500-calorie menu:

Breakfast	1 teaspoon margarine or		
	1 tablespoon light		
	margarine	1 fat	45
Lunch	Add 2 ounces flaked tuna		
	to tuna salad	2 VL protein†	70
	½ grapefruit	1 fruit	60
Dinner	½ cup vegetable rice pilaf	½ starch	40
		1 vegetable	25
	2 teaspoons olive oil for		
	vinaigrette dressing	2 fat	90
		TOTAL	**1,800**

---

†*VL protein = very lean protein*

❖ WEDNESDAY / 1,200 CALORIES ❖

MEAL	MENU	COMPOSITION	CALORIES
Breakfast	1 cup vegetable juice	2 vegetable	50
	½ cup All-Bran cereal	1 starch	80
	1 cup skim milk	1 milk	90
			220
Lunch	1 serving zesty chicken salad*	3 protein	165
		1 vegetable	25
	Small (mini) whole-wheat pita	1 starch	80
	2 cups vegetable salad*	2 vegetable	50
	1 teaspoon olive oil	1 fat	45
	Balsamic vinegar	—	—
			365
Snack	1½ cups chocolate shake*	1 milk	90
Dinner	4 ounces tangy sole*	4 VL protein†	140
	½ cup cooked lima beans	1 starch	80
	1 teaspoon margarine or 1 tablespoon light margarine	1 fat	45
	1 cup spinach	2 vegetable	50
	3 cups vegetable salad*	3 vegetable	75
	Balsamic vinegar	—	—
	½ medium grapefruit	1 fruit	60
			450
Snack	Fresh orange	1 fruit	60
		TOTAL	**1,185**

Recipe is provided in Chapter 13.
†*VL protein = very lean protein*

For a 1,500-calorie menu, add:

Snack	1 cup fresh strawberries	1 fruit	60
Dinner	3 ounces broiled sole	3 protein	105
	½ cup cooked lima beans	1 starch	80
	1 teaspoon olive oil	1 fat	45
		TOTAL	**1,475**

For an 1,800-calorie menu, add to 1,500-calorie menu:

Breakfast	½ cup All-Bran cereal	1 starch	80
Lunch	Add 1 ounce chicken to zesty chicken salad	1 protein	55
	8 large black olives	1 fat	45
	Fresh apple	1 fruit	60
Snack	1 cup plain or artificially sweetened nonfat yogurt	1 milk	90
		TOTAL	**1,805**

❖ THURSDAY / 1,200 CALORIES ❖

MEAL	MENU	COMPOSITION	CALORIES
Breakfast	1 cup V-8 juice	2 vegetable	50
	½ cup oatmeal	1 starch	80
	½ cup skim milk	½ milk	45
	1 teaspoon margarine or 1 tablespoon light margarine	1 fat	45
	1 cup cubed cantaloupe	1 fruit	60
			280
Lunch	1 serving chef's salad*	2 VL protein†	70
		1 protein	55
		3 vegetable	75
	1½ teaspoons Dijon dressing*	1 fat	45
	2 bread sticks	1 starch	80
			325
Snack	¼ cup one-percent-fat cottage cheese	½ milk	45
	Fresh orange	1 fruit	60
			105
Dinner	3 ounces honey-mustard chicken*	3 protein	165
	½ cup peas	1 starch	80
	1 cup cooked cauliflower	2 vegetable	50
	2 cups mixed salad greens with tomato slices	2 vegetable	50
	2 tablespoons fat-free salad dressing	—	25
			370
Snack	1 cup frozen yogurt*	1 milk	90
		½ fruit	30
			120
		TOTAL	**1,200**

―――――――――

Recipe is provided in Chapter 13.

†*VL protein = very lean protein*

For a 1,500-calorie menu, add:

Dinner	Add 2 ounces skinless, boneless chicken breast to honey-mustard chicken	2 protein	110
	½ cup peas	1 starch	80
	1 teaspoon olive oil	1 fat	45
Snack	1 cup cubed honeydew melon	1 fruit	60
		TOTAL	**1,495**

For an 1,800-calorie menu, add to 1,500-calorie menu:

Breakfast	2 slices light whole-grain toast	1 starch	80
Lunch	Add 2 ounces turkey breast to chef's salad	2 VL protein[†]	70
	Fresh orange	1 fruit	60
Dinner	1 teaspoon olive oil	1 fat	45
		TOTAL	**1,750**

[†]VL protein = very lean protein

❖ FRIDAY / 1,200 CALORIES ❖

MEAL	MENU	COMPOSITION	CALORIES
Breakfast	2 slices light whole-grain toast	1 starch	80
	1 teaspoon margarine or 1 tablespoon light margarine	1 fat	45
	½ cup one-percent-fat cottage cheese	1 milk	90
			215
Lunch	Low-calorie microwave meal	2½ protein	140
		2 vegetable	50
		1 starch	80
	1 cup steamed spinach	2 vegetable	50
	2 cups vegetable salad*	2 vegetable	50
	Balsamic vinegar	—	—
			370
Snack	1 slice whole-grain toast	1 starch	80
	1 slice fat-free cheese	½ milk	45
			125
Dinner	3 ounces lean steak	3 protein	165
	1 cup pasta primavera*	1 starch	80
		1 vegetable	25
		½ milk	45
		½ fat	25
	2 cups vegetable salad*	2 vegetable	50
	Balsamic vinegar	—	—
	Fresh apple	1 fruit	60
			450
Snack	1½ cups chocolate shake*	1 milk	90
		TOTAL	**1,250**

Recipe is provided in Chapter 13.

For a 1,500-calorie menu, add:

Breakfast	1 egg and 2 egg whites, scrambled	1 VL protein†	35
		1 medium-fat protein	75
Lunch	Small (mini) whole-wheat pita	1 starch	80
	1 teaspoon margarine or 1 tablespoon light margarine	1 fat	45
	½ medium grapefruit	1 fruit	60
		TOTAL	*1,545*

For an 1,800-calorie menu, add to 1,500-calorie menu:

Dinner	2 ounces lean steak	2 protein	110
	1 cup pasta primavera	1 starch	80
		1 vegetable	25
		½ milk	45
		½ fat	25
		TOTAL	*1,830*

----

†*VL protein = very lean protein*

◆ SATURDAY / 1,200 CALORIES ◆

MEAL	MENU	COMPOSITION	CALORIES
Breakfast	1 cup plain or artificially sweetened nonfat yogurt	1 milk	90
	Fresh orange	1 fruit	60
			150
Lunch	1 serving tuna salad*	3 VL protein†	105
		1 fat	45
		1 vegetable	25
	Small (mini) whole-wheat pita	1 starch	80
	3 cups vegetable salad*	3 vegetable	75
	1½ tablespoons low-calorie vinaigrette	1 fat	45
			375
Snack	1 cup skim milk	1 milk	90
Dinner	4 ounces tangy sole*	4 VL protein†	140
	⅔ cup barley	2 starch	160
	3 cups vegetable salad*	3 vegetable	75
	1½ tablespoons low-calorie vinaigrette*	1 fat	45
	1 cup steamed broccoli with lemon	2 vegetable	50
			470
Snack	Fresh peach	1 fruit	60
	1 cup reduced-fat hot cocoa	½ milk	45
			105
		TOTAL	**1,190**

Recipe is provided in Chapter 13.
†*VL protein = very lean protein*

For a 1,500-calorie menu, add:

Breakfast	½ cup Wheatena	1 starch	80
	1 teaspoon margarine	1 fat	45
Dinner	3 ounces tangy sole	3 VL protein†	105
	1 teaspoon olive oil	1 fat	45
		TOTAL	**1,465**

For an 1,800-calorie menu, add to 1,500-calorie menu:

Breakfast	½ cup Wheatena	1 starch	80
Lunch	Add 1 ounce flaked tuna to tuna salad	1 VL protein†	35
	½ medium grapefruit	1 fruit	60
Snack	4 whole-grain fat-free crackers	½ starch	40
	Fresh apple	1 fruit	60
Dinner	8 large black olives	1 fat	45
		TOTAL	**1,785**

---

†*VL protein = very lean protein*

❖ SUNDAY / 1,200 CALORIES ❖

MEAL	MENU	COMPOSITION	CALORIES
Breakfast	1 cup V-8 juice	2 vegetable	50
	2-egg-white omelette	2 VL protein†	35
	½ cup cooked peppers/ onions	1 vegetable	25
	2 slices light whole-grain toast	1 starch	80
	1 teaspoon margarine or 1 tablespoon light margarine	1 fat	45
			235
Lunch	3 ounces water-packed flaked salmon	3 protein	165
	3 cups vegetable salad*	3 vegetable	75
	1½ tablespoons apple-cider dressing*	—	—
	½ grapefruit	1 fruit	60
	Small (mini) whole-wheat pita	1 starch	80
			380
Snack	1 cup skim milk	1 milk	90
Dinner	1 cup turkey chili*	3 protein	165
		1 vegetable	25
		2 starch	160
	2 cups vegetable salad*	2 vegetable	50
	Balsamic vinegar	—	—
			400
Snack	1 cup frozen yogurt*	1 milk	90
		½ fruit	30
			120
		TOTAL	*1,225*

---

*Recipe is provided in Chapter 13.
†VL protein = very lean protein

For a 1,500-calorie menu, add:

Breakfast	1 cup berries	1 fruit	60
Lunch	2 ounces water-packed flaked salmon	2 protein	110
Dinner	⅓ cup cooked brown rice	1 starch	80
	1 teaspoon canola oil	1 fat	45
		TOTAL	**1,520**

For an 1,800-calorie menu, add to 1,500-calorie menu:

Lunch	1 teaspoon olive oil	1 fat	45
Snack	Fresh apple	1 fruit	60
Dinner	½ cup turkey chili	1½ protein	85
		½ vegetable	15
		1 starch	80
		TOTAL	**1,805**

13

RECIPES FOR THE
GETTING HEALTHY PLAN

❖

MAIN COURSES

Pasta Primavera

❖ ❖ ❖

1 tablespoon olive oil
2 shallots, finely diced
2 cloves garlic, minced
3 cups broccoli, cut into small florets
½ cup carrot strips, cut into ½-inch lengths
½ cup zucchini, cut into 1-inch cubes
½ cup yellow squash, cut into 1-inch cubes
1 cup cherry or plum tomatoes
4 tablespoons fresh or 2 tablespoons dried basil
4 teaspoons fresh or 2 teaspoons dried parsley
2 teaspoons dried oregano
¼ teaspoon cayenne pepper flakes (optional)

¼   **cup light ricotta cheese**
½   **cup chicken broth**
½   **pound fusilli pasta**
¼   **cup Parmesan cheese**
     Salt and pepper to taste

In a nonstick skillet, heat olive oil, shallots, and garlic. Add broccoli, carrots, zucchini, and squash. Stir vigorously over high heat until vegetables are lightly cooked but still firm (al dente), about 4 to 6 minutes.

Add tomatoes, basil, parsley, oregano, and pepper flakes. Stir 1 to 2 minutes and remove from heat.

In a food processor, puree ricotta, then add chicken broth.

Cook pasta according to package instructions and drain. Toss vegetables with pasta. Add ricotta mixture. Top with Parmesan cheese. Season with salt and pepper.

Yield: *8 servings*
Serving size: *1 cup*
Calories per serving: *175*
Per-serving composition: *1 starch*
                             1 vegetable
                             ½ milk
                             ½ fat

Meat Sauce for Pasta

❖ ❖ ❖

½ pound extra-lean beef
1 large onion, chopped
2 cloves garlic, minced
1 28-ounce can crushed tomatoes
1 6-ounce can tomato paste (no added salt)
2 teaspoons fresh or 1 teaspoon dried parsley
2 teaspoons fresh or 1 teaspoon dried basil
½ teaspoon oregano
1 cup water
½ teaspoon sugar (optional, if the sauce tastes tart)

Brown beef on one side in a nonstick skillet. Drain any oil from the meat.

Add onion and garlic and continue to brown beef and cook onion until it softens.

Stir in tomatoes, tomato paste, parsley, basil, oregano, and water.

Cook over medium heat and simmer sauce for 20 to 30 minutes.

Yield: 10 servings
Serving size: ½ cup
Calories per serving: 95
Per-serving composition: 1 protein
1½ vegetable

This sauce can also be made without meat:
Calories per ½-cup serving: 50
Per-serving composition: 2 vegetable

Or, you can add 2 ounces shrimp or clams:
Calories per half-cup serving: 90
Per-serving composition: 1 protein
2 vegetable

One-half cup of any of these sauces can be served over 1 cup of cooked pasta, which has 160 calories and counts as 2 starches.

Eggplant Sauce for Pasta

———————— ❖ ❖ ❖ ————————

1	large eggplant, cut into 1-inch cubes
2	onions, sliced
2	cloves garlic, finely minced
1	tablespoon olive oil
⅓	cup dry white wine
1	28-ounce can whole tomatoes
1	15-ounce can tomato sauce
	1 to 2 teaspoons sugar
½	cup fresh mushrooms, sliced
¼	cup Parmesan cheese
2	teaspoons fresh or 1 teaspoon dried basil
2	teaspoons fresh or 1 teaspoon dried oregano
2	teaspoons fresh or 1 teaspoon dried parsley
	Salt and pepper to taste

Using a nonstick pan, combine eggplant, onion, and garlic in olive oil and wine. Cook until eggplant is tender, about 10 minutes.

Stir both cans of tomatoes into the pan and add sugar. Mix in mushrooms, cheese, basil, oregano, and parsley. Break up tomatoes.

Heat to boiling. Reduce heat and simmer about 45 minutes.

Yield: 7 servings
Serving size: 1 cup
Calories per serving: 125
Per-serving composition: ½ protein
3 vegetable
½ fat

One-half cup of this sauce can be served over 1 cup of cooked pasta, which has 160 calories and counts as 2 starches.

Poached Salmon

——————— ◆ ◆ ◆ ———————

1   **pound salmon fillets**
2   **cups water**
¼   **cup white wine**
2   **tablespoons lemon juice**
1   **bay leaf**
1   **small whole onion, cut into quarters**
1   **celery stalk, cut into four pieces**
     Salt and pepper to taste
     Parsley sprigs

Bring water to boil in a shallow pan.

Place salmon in pan. Add wine, celery, onion, lemon juice, and bay leaf. Bring to boil; cover and simmer for 10 to 15 minutes.

Refrigerate and serve cold, seasoned with salt and pepper and garnished with parsley. This dish is delicious when served with yogurt-dill sauce.

Yield: 4 servings
Serving size: 3 ounces
Calories per serving: 190
Per-serving composition: 3 protein
                                            1 vegetable

Tangy Flounder or Sole
❖ ❖ ❖

1¼ pound flounder or sole fillet (⅛ inch to ¼ inch thick)
¼   cup balsamic vinegar
¼   cup lemon juice
1   teaspoon dried mustard powder
1   small yellow onion, chopped
2   teaspoons fresh or 1 teaspoon dried parsley
    Lemon slices (optional)

Rinse and pat dry fish fillets. Place fish in 10-inch by 8-inch ovenproof glass or stainless steel baking dish.

Combine vinegar, lemon juice, dried mustard powder, and chopped onion in small mixing bowl. Pour over fillets.

Cover dish and marinate fish in refrigerator for approximately 2 hours.

Preheat broiler. Remove cover from dish and place dish in broiler for approximately 4 to 6 minutes, or until fish is white and flaky throughout.

Garnish with parsley and lemon slices.

Yield: 4 servings
Serving size: 4 ounces
Calories per serving: 140
Per-serving composition: 4 very lean protein

Chicken Stir-Fry

— ❖ ❖ ❖ —

1   **pound boneless chicken cutlets, cut into 1-inch slices**
⅓   **cup low-sodium soy sauce**
1   **tablespoon grated ginger**
4   **teaspoons olive oil**
3   **cloves crushed garlic**
2   **cups broccoli florets**
1   **cup carrots, thinly sliced**
1   **cup homemade chicken stock or low-sodium bouillon**
1   **cup snow peas**
1   **cup fresh mushrooms, sliced**
1   **cup red or green peppers, sliced into thin strips**
     Salt and pepper to taste

Marinate chicken with soy sauce and ginger for several hours in the refrigerator, stirring occasionally.

In a large nonstick skillet, heat olive oil over medium heat. Add garlic and sauté 2 minutes.

Add chicken with marinade, broccoli, and carrots and cook until chicken loses its pink color. Add chicken broth, snow peas, mushrooms, and peppers. Cover and reduce heat to low. Cook 15 minutes, stirring frequently. Season with salt and pepper.

Yield: 4 servings
Serving size: ¼ of recipe
Calories per serving: 285
Per-serving composition: 3 protein
3 vegetable
1 fat

Turkey Chili

❖ ❖ ❖

1   **pound ground white-meat turkey**
½   **cup chopped onions**
1   **clove garlic, minced**
1   **16-ounce can black beans, rinsed and drained**
1   **16-ounce can red kidney beans, rinsed and drained**
1   **28-ounce can whole tomatoes, undrained and chopped**
     1 to 2 tablespoons chili powder to taste
1   **teaspoon dried oregano**
1   **teaspoon ground cumin**
¼   **teaspoon cayenne pepper (optional)**
     Salt and pepper to taste

Brown turkey with onions and garlic in a nonstick skillet over medium heat. Continue to sauté until meat is no longer pink. Reduce heat and add remaining ingredients; simmer, covered, for 15 to 20 minutes.

Yield: 8 servings
Serving size: 1 cup
Calories per serving: 350
Per-serving composition: 3 protein
                          1 vegetable
                          2 starch

Vegetable Rice Pilaf

———— ◆ ◆ ◆ ————

¾ cup uncooked brown rice
   Vegetable spray (such as Pam)
½ medium red onion, chopped
2 garlic cloves, minced
3 celery stalks, chopped into bite-sized pieces
1 large tomato, chopped
1 large sweet red pepper, sliced into strips
1 large green pepper, sliced into strips
   Black pepper
   Parsley sprigs

Cook rice according to package directions, omitting use of butter, margarine, or oil. While rice is cooking prepare all the vegetables.

Spray a large skillet with vegetable spray. Sauté onion and garlic until tender, about 2 minutes. Add all other vegetables to skillet, sprinkle with black pepper to taste, and continue to cook until tender, about 5 more minutes. Stir occasionally.

Add cooked rice to vegetable blend and stir to combine.

Serve hot, garnished with a sprig of parsley and black pepper.

Yield: 4 servings
Serving size: 1 cup
Calories per serving: 130
Per-serving composition: 1 starch
*   2 vegetable*

Zesty Chicken Salad

❖ ❖ ❖

¼	cup balsamic vinegar
2	tablespoons lemon juice
1	teaspoon dried mustard powder
1	teaspoon dried oregano
3	ounces skinless, boneless chicken breast, cooked and cubed
1	medium tomato, chopped
1	large lettuce leaf

Combine vinegar, lemon juice, mustard powder, and oregano in a small mixing bowl. Place chicken and tomato in another bowl. Pour vinegar marinade over chicken and tomato. Cover and refrigerate for 1 hour or more.

Serve cold chicken on top of lettuce leaf. This salad is equally tasty with turkey.

Yield: 1 serving
Calories per serving: 190
Per-serving composition: 3 protein
                                      1 vegetable

Chicken Tarragon

❖ ❖ ❖

1	**pound skinless, boneless chicken breasts**
¼	**cup chicken broth**
¼	**cup lemon juice**
1	**teaspoon dried mustard powder**
2	**tablespoons fresh or 1 tablespoon dried tarragon**
⅛	**teaspoon black pepper**

Cut away all visible fat from chicken.

Mix broth, lemon juice, mustard powder, tarragon, and pepper in a small bowl.

Place chicken breasts in a glass baking dish. Pour liquid/herb mixture over chicken. Cover and marinate at least 2 hours or overnight in the refrigerator.

Bake in preheated 325°F oven for 25 to 30 minutes, or until cooked through.

Yield: 4 servings
Serving size: 3 ounces
Calories per serving: 165
Per-serving composition: 3 protein

Honey-Mustard Chicken

————— ❖ ❖ ❖ —————

1½   tablespoons Dijon or raspberry mustard
1   tablespoon honey
     Pepper to taste
1   pound skinless, boneless chicken breasts, flattened or
       thinly sliced
     Vegetable spray (such as Pam)

Mix together mustard, honey, and pepper. Coat each piece of chicken with this mixture. Cover and marinate in the refrigerator for at least 1 hour (the longer the better).

Spray a skillet with vegetable spray and sauté the chicken, turning occasionally, until it is browned on both sides and cooked through. Cooking time is just 5 to 10 minutes.

Yield: 4 servings
Serving size: 3 ounces
Calories per serving: 165
Per-serving composition: 3 protein

Chicken Dijon

❖ ❖ ❖

4   skinless, boneless chicken breasts, flattened
¼   cup Dijon mustard
½   cup dry vermouth or white wine
1   tablespoon lemon juice
    Fresh ground pepper to taste
    Dried tarragon, crushed

Place chicken breasts side by side in bottom of shallow, oven-proof baking dish.

Blend mustard, wine, lemon juice, and ground pepper in mixing bowl and pour over chicken breasts. Sprinkle with tarragon.

Cover chicken and marinate for several hours or overnight in the refrigerator.

Preheat broiler. Remove chicken from marinade and place on rack in broiler pan about 6 inches from heat for 5 minutes on each side or until tender.

Baste frequently with additional marinade.

Yield: 4 servings
Serving size: 3 ounces
Calories per serving: 165
Per-serving composition: 3 protein

SALADS AND SIDE DISHES

Tuna Salad

1   3½ ounce can water-packed tuna
1   tablespoon reduced-fat mayonnaise
1   celery stalk, chopped
1   scallion, chopped
1   teaspoon red-wine vinegar
    Pepper and garlic powder to taste

Drain tuna, mix all ingredients together, and stir well.

Yield: 1 serving
Calories per serving: 175
Per-serving composition: 3 very lean protein
                          1 fat
                          1 vegetable

Chef's Salad

❖ ❖ ❖

2   cups torn romaine leaves
½   medium-sized tomato, cut into wedges
½   green pepper, sliced
1   carrot, sliced
½   cup cucumber, sliced
2   ounces cooked skinless turkey breast, cut into 1-inch strips
1   ounce cooked lean roast beef, cut into 1-inch strips
    Fresh ground pepper to taste

Mix all vegetable ingredients together. Sprinkle turkey and roast beef strips on top and season with pepper. Serve with any of the dressings on pages 217–220.

Yield: 1 serving
Calories per serving: 200
Per-serving composition: 2 very lean protein, 1 lean protein
*   3 vegetable*

Vegetable Salad

❖ ❖ ❖

1	cup torn romaine leaves
1	cup torn green- or red-leaf lettuce
1	medium tomato, sliced
½	red pepper, sliced
1	large carrot, sliced
5	fresh mushrooms, sliced
½	cucumber, sliced
1	tablespoon chopped onion
	Fresh ground pepper to taste

Put all ingredients into large wooden salad bowl and toss. Serve with any of the dressings on pages 217–220.

Yield: 4 servings
Serving size: 1 cup
Calories per serving: 25
Per-serving composition: 1 vegetable

Bulgur

❖ ❖ ❖

1   **cup uncooked bulgur**
1   **cup water**
1   **cup chicken broth**
1   **teaspoon canola oil**
1   **teaspoon onion powder**
1   **teaspoon garlic powder**
2   **tablespoons fresh or 1 tablespoon dried parsley**

In a medium pan, mix all ingredients together. Cover and bring to boil over medium heat. Reduce heat and simmer 15 to 20 minutes, or until all liquid is absorbed.

Yield: 8 servings
Serving size: ⅓ cup, cooked
Calories per serving: 80
Per-serving composition: 1 starch

Cottage Fries

❖ ❖ ❖

    Vegetable spray (such as Pam)
2   unpeeled medium potatoes (6 ounces each), washed
      and thinly sliced
    Garlic powder
    Paprika
    Salt to taste

Spray a baking dish with vegetable spray and arrange the potatoes in a single layer. Sprinkle generously with garlic and paprika and add salt if desired.

Bake at 400°F for 10 to 15 minutes, turn potatoes over, and cook for another 10 to 15 minutes, or until they are lightly browned.

Yield: 4 servings
Serving size: ¼ of recipe
Calories per serving: 80
Per-serving composition: 1 starch

DRESSINGS

Low-Calorie Vinaigrette

❖ ❖ ❖

2 tablespoons olive oil
3 tablespoons balsamic vinegar
3 tablespoons rice vinegar
¼ teaspoon salt
Pepper and garlic to taste

Combine all ingredients in a small bowl and whisk together. Or, you can put all ingredients in a glass jar, cover, and shake vigorously until well blended. Serve on salads, or raw or cooked vegetables.

Yield: ½ cup
Serving size: 1½ tablespoons
Calories per serving: 45
Per-serving composition: 1 fat

Dijon Dressing

❖ ❖ ❖

2	tablespoons vegetable oil
6	tablespoons red wine vinegar
2	garlic cloves, minced
2	tablespoons Dijon mustard

Combine all ingredients in a small bowl and whisk together. Or, you can put all ingredients in a glass jar, cover, and shake vigorously until well blended. Serve on salad, raw or cooked vegetables, or chicken.

Yield: ¼ *cup*
Serving size: 1½ *tablespoons*
Calories per serving: 45
Per-serving composition: 1 *fat*

Lemon-Yogurt Dressing

❖ ❖ ❖

½ cup plain nonfat yogurt
1 lemon, finely chopped zest and juice
½ garlic clove, minced
¼ teaspoon chopped fresh or ⅛ teaspoon dried parsley
Pepper to taste

Combine all ingredients in a small bowl and whisk together. Or, you can put all ingredients in a glass jar, cover, and shake vigorously until well blended.

Delicious with salads or with poached, broiled, or grilled poultry or fish.

Yield: ½ cup
Serving size: 1 tablespoon
Calories per serving: 10

Apple-Cider Dressing

——————— ❖ ❖ ❖ ———————

¼   cup apple cider vinegar
3   tablespoons lemon juice
2   teaspoons artificial sweetener
1   teaspoon dried mustard powder
1   teaspoon whole celery seed

Combine all ingredients in a small bowl and whisk together. Or, you can put all ingredients in a glass jar, cover, and shake vigorously until well blended. Refrigerate for at least 1 hour for best results.

Yield: ½ cup
Serving size: 1½ tablespoons
Calories per serving: Fewer than 5

Yogurt Dill Sauce
for Poached Salmon

❖ ❖ ❖

1   cup plain nonfat yogurt
1   teaspoon Dijon mustard
2   tablespoons fresh dill

Mix mustard with yogurt. Chop dill; add to yogurt mixture.

Yield: 1 cup/16 servings
Serving size: 1 tablespoon
Calories per serving: 5

SNACKS AND DESSERTS

Spinach-Yogurt Dip

❖ ❖ ❖

1   package (10 ounces) frozen spinach, chopped
½   cup plain nonfat yogurt
1   cup nonfat sour cream
1   package Knorrs dried vegetable soup mix

Drain spinach well. Mix with yogurt and sour cream. Slowly stir in dried soup mix. (This recipe can also be made without the spinach.)

Yield: 8 servings
Serving size: ¼ cup
Calories per serving: 35
Per-serving composition: ¼ milk
*   ½ vegetable*

Chocolate Shake

❖ ❖ ❖

1   cup skim milk
½   cup diet chocolate soda
5   ice cubes
¼   teaspoon cinnamon

Place all ingredients in blender and blend for 1 minute.

Yield: 1 serving
Serving size: 1½ cups
Calories per serving: 90
Per-serving composition: 1 milk

Frozen Yogurt

❖ ❖ ❖

2 **cups nonfat plain yogurt**
½ **cup mixed fresh fruit**
   Cinnamon to taste
   Artificial sweetener to taste

Empty contents of container of nonfat plain yogurt into a cone-style coffee filter. Place the filter over a wide-mouthed jar and place in the refrigerator overnight.

Pour the drained yogurt into a bowl and flavor with the fresh fruit, cinnamon, and artificial sweetener. Add low-fat hot chocolate powder if you like. Stir well.

Pour into a plastic container and freeze for at least 12 hours.

This is a great substitute for commercial frozen yogurt, which often is laden with fats and sugar.

Yield: 2 cups
Serving size: 1 cup
Calories per serving: 120
Per-serving composition: 1 milk
                          ½ fruit

14

ADDING VARIETY
TO YOUR DIET

❖

The food exchanges and recipe substitutions in this chapter allow you to eat only what you enjoy. Using the information here, you can modify the Getting Healthy menu plans or create your own. You can also transform a high-fat recipe into an ideal weight control food. And you'll find a slew of ideas for adding flavor to your food without fat or calories.

THE EXCHANGE PRINCIPLE

One serving of any food on the following list can be exchanged for one serving of any other food, as long as the listed portion size is equivalent. Each food has the same calorie count and the same number of carbohydrate, fat, and protein grams. For example, a cup of skim milk can be exchanged for the same amount of nonfat yogurt. A small baked potato substitutes for a serving of lentils. You can eat veal roast instead of pork tenderloin, tuna fish rather than chicken breast, an ear of corn in lieu of green peas.

Study the options presented here and you will discover an almost infinite list of food choices.

Protein / Very Lean, Lean, and Medium-Fat Meat and Meat Substitutes

The very lean proteins have approximately 35 calories and 1 gram of fat per one-ounce serving.

Fresh turkey, white meat, no skin; processed, skinless turkey breast

Fish: fresh or frozen cod, flounder, sole, haddock, halibut

Tuna (canned in water)

Shellfish: clams, crab, lobster, scallops, shrimp, imitation shellfish

Fat-free cheeses (35–45 calories per ounce, can be exchanged for milk)

Egg whites (2 whites = 1 ounce protein)

Egg substitutes (¼ cup = 1 ounce protein)

The lean proteins have approximately 55 calories and 2–3 grams of fat per one-ounce serving.

Chicken breast, skin removed

Turkey, dark meat, or ground turkey meat

Any other fresh, frozen, or canned water-packed fish not listed above

Lean red meats, all visible fat removed (no more than once or twice a week)

 Beef: flank, round, sirloin, or tenderloin

 Lamb: roast, leg, loin cuts, or loin select

 Veal: chops or roast

 Pork: fresh ham, tenderloin

 Luncheon meats: lean ham, turkey pastrami, or other low-fat processed meats with 3 grams or less of fat per ounce

Low-fat cheeses with less than 3 grams of fat per ounce

One-percent-fat cottage cheese (also listed in milk group); ½ cup can be counted as 2 ounces of protein = 90 calories if used in a meal as a protein equivalent.

On occasion, a medium-fat meat could be used, but no more than 3 servings per week.

The medium-fat proteins have approximately 75 calories and 5 grams of fat per one-ounce serving.

Tofu (4 ounces or ½ cup, a heart-healthy choice which can be used without restriction)

1 medium egg
Beef (any prime cut such as prime rib)

Starch/Bread

80 calories per serving, as listed below

These foods are listed from the lowest glycemic index to the highest; for people using Menu Plan II, lower is better, with the top seven choices being the best. When selecting a vegetarian meal, you may count 1 cup of legumes as 2 starch/bread and 2 lean meat servings.

⅓ cup legumes (dried beans, lentils, split peas)
½ cup cooked green peas, corn, or lima beans
½ cup cooked pasta, ⅓ cup barley, bulgur, or couscous
½ cup yam or sweet potato
½ cup bran cereal (All-Bran, Fiber One)
1 slice pumpernickel or whole-grain bread
2 slices light pumpernickel or whole-grain bread
Small (mini) pita bread
6-inch ear of corn
⅓ cup cooked rice
3 cups air-popped or microwave popcorn with no fat
4 melba toast
4–8 fat-free crackers (¾ ounce)
2 rice cakes
¼ ounce pretzels
¼ cup unsweetened flaked cereal
½ cup bran flakes or shredded wheat
1 small baked potato (3 ounces)

Fruits

60 calories per serving

These foods are listed from the lowest glycemic index to the highest; for people using Menu Plan II, lower is better, with the top five choices being the best.
1 cup berries
½ medium grapefruit

1 small apple, orange, or medium peach
2 small tangerines
1 cup cubed melon
½ cup fresh fruit salad
½ small banana or 1 small pear
12 large cherries
17 small grapes
½ cup fruit juice (use infrequently)

Vegetables

25 calories per serving

½ cup cooked vegetables
½ cup vegetable juice
1 cup raw vegetables
1 cup salad greens (including endive, lettuce, spinach)

Milk

90 to 110 calories per serving

1 cup skim milk
1 cup one-percent-fat milk
½ cup evaporated skim milk
1 cup plain or artificially sweetened nonfat yogurt
½ cup nonfat or one-percent-fat cottage cheese (can be
    exchanged for lean meat)
2 ounces (approximately 2 slices) nonfat or low-fat cheese with
    less than 3 grams of fat per ounce (can be exchanged for lean
    meat)

Fat

45 calories per serving

1 teaspoon oil (preferably olive or canola)
1 tablespoon reduced-fat margarine
1 tablespoon reduced-fat butter
1 teaspoon margarine
1 teaspoon butter
1 tablespoon reduced-fat (light) mayonnaise

1 tablespoon regular salad dressing
1 tablespoon cream cheese
⅛ medium avocado
8 large black olives or 10 stuffed green olives

RECIPE SUBSTITUTIONS

Another way to modify your diet is to alter the recipes in conventional cookbooks. As a general rule, you can cut the suggested fat or salt in half without losing much flavor. When you bake, substitute low-fat yogurt or applesauce for any fat you remove to maintain moistness. In main dishes, wine, lemon juice, salsa, balsamic vinegar, and seasonings will tenderize most meats and flavor foods, often reducing the need for fat or salt.

Here are some other suggestions for turning a high-calorie, high-fat, or high-sodium recipe into one that is right for a Getting Healthy eater:

If the recipe calls for	Substitute	Result
1 cup whole milk	1 cup skim milk	Reduce calories by 60
½ cup sour cream	½ cup low-fat cottage cheese, puréed in a blender or food processor	120 fewer calories and 19 grams less fat
2 whole eggs	1 whole egg and 2 egg whites	200 milligrams less cholesterol and 50 fewer calories
4 tablespoons butter	2 tablespoons vegetable oil	132 milligrams less cholesterol and 270 fewer calories
1 cup heavy cream	1 cup one-percent-fat milk	Cut fat by 86 grams, calories by 730

If the recipe calls for	Substitute	Result
1 teaspoon salt	½ teaspoon salt	Reduce sodium by 1,000 milligrams
1 cup instant broth	1 cup home-made or unsalted bouillon	Reduce sodium by 800 to 1,200 milligrams
1 cup sugar	½ cup sugar	Reduce calories by 480

LOW-FAT AND FAT-FREE FOODS

You can also eat more balanced and nutritious food by getting in the habit of reading food labels and purchasing low-fat and fat-free products. In recent years, many of these foods have entered the market, greatly reducing the need to use their fattier cousins. For example, traditional mayonnaise has 11 grams of fat per tablespoon while light mayonnaise has just 5 grams; the prize-winner is nonfat mayonnaise, with less than 1 fat gram. Look on the supermarket shelves for fat-free desserts, dairy products, frozen foods, and canned goods.

Keep in mind that while it is great to lower your fat consumption, calories still count—don't go overboard just because a product is labeled fat-free. And be sure to read the labels carefully because total calorie counts vary from one product to another.

Here are a few examples of easy substitutions to take fat and calories out of your diet:

- ◆ Use fat-free salad dressing. (Save between 20 and 70 calories per tablespoon compared to traditional dressing.)
- ◆ Eat water-packed tuna. (Save 70 calories and 7 fat grams per small can [2.7 ounces] compared to oil-packed tuna.)

❖ Eat a baked potato with fat-free sour cream. (Save 130 calories per serving compared to french fries.)

❖ Eat turkey, lean ham, or some of the other low-fat meats on the market. (Save 150 to 200 calories per serving compared to ordinary luncheon meats.)

❖ Use jelly on your toast, preferably all-fruit jelly. (Save 50 to 100 calories and 11 grams of fat per tablespoon compared to butter.)

❖ Use nonfat sour cream. (Save 40 calories and 5 grams of fat per 2-tablespoon serving compared to ordinary sour cream.)

❖ Use fat-free cream cheese. (Save 75 calories and 10 grams of fat per 2-tablespoon serving compared to ordinary cream cheese.)

There are also some scrumptious, low-fat desserts that satisfy your sweet tooth without blowing your diet to pieces:

❖ Angel-food cake with fresh fruit. (Save at least 100 calories per 2-ounce slice over regular iced cake.)

❖ Baked apple with fruit juice and cinnamon. (Save at least 100 calories over a candy bar.)

❖ Fresh or frozen fruits, such as bananas, grapes, or berries. (Save 200 calories per serving over ice cream.)

❖ Ginger snaps, vanilla wafers, or Fig Newtons. (Save approximately 20% calories per serving over most other cookies.)

SEASONING YOUR FOOD

Seasoning your foods with fresh herbs, spices, bouillon, and citrus juice instead of butter, oil, and salt is another painless way to save fat calories and add pizzazz. You can use them in any combination and in any quantity you wish—the only restrictions are your personal preferences, your taste, and your imagination.

I prefer using fresh herbs when they are available. Although it takes a little more work to prepare them, it is well worth the added flavor. If you do purchase seasonings in the supermarket, be sure to read the label first so that you can avoid the sodium or salt that some manufacturers unnecessarily add to their products.

Other condiments that give your food added flavor without adding many calories include:

All-fruit jelly

Horseradish

Lemon juice

Lime juice

Mustard

Salsa

Vinegar

Generally, I use more seasonings than the recipes suggest—typically, I will double the amount, and sometimes throw in an extra handful beyond that, just for good measure. The calorie counts for herbs and spices are very low or nonexistent. It is a good idea to use a light hand with the spicier condiments, such as horseradish and salsa, until you become accustomed to their strong flavor.

Many types of flavored vinegar are sold in local supermarkets these days. Each vinegar has its own special character and, like a good wine, is well matched with particular kinds of food. Experiment to find out what you enjoy. For example, balsamic vinegar is hearty and delicious on salads while the delicate Japanese rice vinegar is a lovely addition to fish dishes. Many people like fruity or herbal vinegars on chicken.

By the way, adding a little bit of salt is not illegal in my book and it brings out flavor in many foods. As long as you don't have a blood pressure problem and you aren't eating too many processed foods, which tend to be high in salt, a little bit of added salt should present no problem. Taste your food first, though, and remember, moderation is the key.

PART FIVE

THE EXERCISE PROGRAM

15

BASIC EXERCISE PRINCIPLES

❖

Exercising is just as important to weight control as eating properly. While it is possible to lose weight without exercising, it is almost impossible to keep it off unless you are physically active.

There is a great deal of research documenting the link between exercise and long-term weight maintenance. One dramatic study was conducted in 1989 within the Boston Police Department. Dieting police officers were divided into two groups: One group added an exercise program to their diet while the other did not. At first, both groups lost weight at approximately the same rate. After their weight goals were met, researchers continued to monitor the participants and 18 months later made this startling discovery: Police officers who were exercising regularly maintained weight loss while those who had not been physically active regained almost all the weight they had shed.

Some people cannot let go of the idea that exercise is a dirty word. If you hold a mental image of sweaty bodies and slick, competitive health clubs in your head, it is no small wonder that you are turned off or intimidated by exercise. The first thing you have to do is let go of that stereotype. Exercise helps you look good, feel good, and live longer. The key to making it a regular habit is to find an activity you enjoy. The demands of the Getting Healthy plan are modest—when you first begin to exercise, all I ask is that you get moving. Any physical activity is better than no activity at all. You can start by walking around the block. If you normally take public transportation, get off one stop earlier than you usually do and walk the rest of the way. Climb the last two flights of stairs to your office instead of taking the elevator. Even some gentle stretching while you are watching television helps you become more limber, laying the foundation on which you can build more exercise.

Take it slow and easy at first. Gradually, you will begin to see how much better you feel. You will begin to notice that you have an extra degree of control over your weight. It won't be long before you are ready for a more rigorous workout. The more room you make for exercise in your daily life, the sooner you'll discover how much better it can make you feel.

WHAT EXERCISE DOES FOR YOU

You need to do two different types of exercise in order to control your weight: aerobic exercises and resistance exercises. Weight-bearing aerobic activities, such as walking, jogging, and bicycle riding, build endurance and increase the amount of oxygen-rich hemoglobin in your bloodstream, which helps the cardiovascular system to operate more efficiently. As a result, your body is better able to burn the fuel you consume in the form of fats and carbohydrates. Resistance exercises, such as weight lifting, build muscle tissue and enhance your physical strength.

You can reap all of the weight control benefits of exercise with a modest effort. As little as 20 minutes of aerobic exercise as often as possible and 20 minutes more of resistance exercises every other day is all you need, although more is better. Exactly how you schedule your exercise sessions is up to you. Some people prefer to alternate aerobic and resistance exercises while others prefer to do both workouts in the same day. As long as you develop, and stick with, a regular program, the details are up to you.

The Physical Benefits

Here is what exercise can do for your body:

- ◆ Increase your metabolic rate, helping you to burn more calories.
- ◆ Counter the reduced state.
- ◆ Lower your body's insulin levels.
- ◆ Maintain a lower blood pressure and cholesterol count.
- ◆ Reduce the LPL enzyme level on your fat cells and increase it on your muscle cells, allowing you to store fewer calories as fat.
- ◆ Improve your waist-to-hip ratio.
- ◆ Increase muscle mass and possibly stimulate the production of as-yet unknown enzymes in the muscles that apparently prevent weight regain.
- ◆ Increase your body's ability to use oxygen.
- ◆ Help you discover your own strength.
- ◆ Help you get more in tune with your body, making it easier to make wise food choices.

The Mental Benefits

Here is what exercise can do for your mind:

- ◆ Improve your concentration.
- ◆ Help you stay focused on your diet.
- ◆ Help you avoid lapsing into old eating habits.
- ◆ Prevent you from becoming breathless so readily.
- ◆ Make you look better and feel better.
- ◆ Build a positive mental attitude.
- ◆ Alleviate your fear of challenging physical tasks.

Within four or five weeks of exercising regularly, you will begin to notice significant physiological changes. You will feel stronger both because you are building muscle mass and because you are reeducating the nerve pathways that send signals between your brain and your muscles. If you have been sedentary, those pathways have been stagnant; as you begin working out, the pathways become more polished, and you'll feel much more alert.

Activity breeds activity. The stronger you become, the more enthusiastic you will be about physical challenges.

EXCUSES THAT WON'T WASH

When it comes to exercising, I've heard just about every excuse in the book. And frankly, I don't think too much of them. Here are some of the claims that I have heard—and the truth about each one.

Exercise increases my appetite.

Studies have actually shown that overweight people are less likely than leaner people to get hungry after exercise, possibly because they have more reserve energy upon which to draw. If you feel the urge to eat after a workout, add a healthy post-workout snack, such as a piece of fruit, to your daily meal plan. You may also want to experiment with different schedules. Some people feel ravenous all day if they exercise in the morning whereas others discover that morning exercise curbs their appetite for the rest of the day. Find out what works for you.

I'll gain weight when I build muscles.

Not necessarily. It is possible to build muscle mass and lose weight at the same time. At first, you may add a few pounds of muscle, but you'll soon be burning more than enough fat to compensate. When you start exercising, don't worry too much about what the scale says. As you get in shape, your shrinking waistline will demonstrate the benefits of physical fitness.

I don't have time to exercise.

Sure you do. We're all busy, but there are ways to squeeze exercise into any schedule using a technique I call "leveraging time." Say, for example, a bus trip across town normally takes 20 minutes. You might be able to walk that same distance in 35 minutes.

By adding only 15 minutes to your travel time, you have given yourself 35 minutes of exercise. Or, you can park at the far end of the local mall. The walk between your car and the shops takes no longer than the time you would have spent driving around searching for a more convenient spot.

It is too late for me to get in shape.
No matter what your age or fitness level, it is never too late to improve your health and your body's ability to win at weight control with exercise. Walk rapidly for just 30 minutes a day, three or four times a week, and you may eventually turn your biological clock back 10 years. Regular aerobic activity may reduce your risk of a heart attack dramatically. No matter how sedentary you have been, it is possible to exercise enough to increase your muscular strength, flexibility, cardiovascular function, and even your ability to process information.

I get burned out from exercise.
I admit that it is possible to become sick and tired of exercise. You may feel fatigued or just plain bored. Although most people have more energy once they begin to exercise regularly, the obligation to set aside time for a workout, week in and week out, may eventually make you feel irritable and rebellious. If you become thoroughly fed up, you may even stop exercising altogether.

Try to add variety to your routine if you start to feel resentful about it. You might want to change the type of exercise you are doing, or the time and place that you do it. It may even be appropriate to take a break altogether. Making a conscious decision to call "time out" for a few days—and scheduling a workout for a specific time afterward—is much wiser than letting weeks slip by without any exercise at all.

I'm embarrassed by the way I look.
Many people don't want to exercise in public because they are self-conscious about their bodies. There are plenty of healthy ways to work out that can be done in the privacy of your own home. This attitude highlights the very reason exercise is so important—you are obviously in dire need of improving your body image and getting in closer touch with yourself.

HEALTH CLUBS AND PERSONAL TRAINERS

The Getting Healthy exercise program is designed to be used in many ways: You can follow the instructions by yourself, enlist a friend to share the experience, or seek the expert help of a professional fitness trainer. Some people prefer to work out alone whereas others need the motivation that a health club membership can provide.

Finding a Health Club

If you plan to get most of your exercise from walking or other outdoor activities, a health club may not be necessary, but being surrounded by other fitness freaks can be a plus. You may also enjoy some of the pampering attached to many health clubs—a sauna, steam room, and massage are often available. Health club prices run anywhere from a few hundred dollars a year to well over $1,000. Many also charge a one-time initiation fee. Check to see if there are additional fees for the services you want.

Make sure the health club you choose is conveniently located to your office or home. Even the best facility is worthless if you don't use it. Most clubs will give you a tour or a free voucher to use the facility on a one-day trial basis.

Here is what else you should look for before plunking down any cash:

❖ Find out if there are special programs targeted at overweight people.

❖ Find out how busy the club is. Try to stop by at the time you expect to do most of your exercising.

❖ Look at the equipment. Do they have the machines you like? Is there enough variety?

❖ Ask what kind of classes are available.

❖ Make sure the club is clean.

❖ Sit in on a class or talk to some of the instructors. Are they understanding and helpful? Or pushy and condescending? You are entitled to work with someone who is patient and understands that you will progress slowly.

❖ If you have children, ask if child care is available. Take a look at the facilities and make sure you will feel comfortable leaving your child there.

❖ Talk to patrons in the locker room and ask whether they are satisfied.

❖ Read the membership contract carefully before signing. You should have the right to cancel and get a full refund for at least a few days after signing up.

About Personal Trainers

Another option to consider is one-to-one instruction from a personal trainer or fitness expert. Some professionals will come to your home; others make their services available at an hourly rate at health clubs and local Y's. By monitoring your exercise routines, demonstrating techniques, and providing motivation, trainers often provide an extra push to help you get started and to stick with your commitment. Just the act of scheduling an appointment with a trainer greatly increases the chances that you'll actually exercise.

To find someone who can help, call the fitness clubs in your community or contact the Aerobics and Fitness Association of America for a referral (see Resources). Your instructor doesn't have to be a muscle-bound model in order to help. To the contrary, an instructor who is familiar with the special needs of overweight people may be the best choice for you. Talk to a number of different candidates for the job before making your selection. Explain what you are looking for and make sure they are responsive to your needs. Don't work with instructors who bully or intimidate you. Remember, exercise should be fun!

KEEPING AT IT

Here are some tips to keep you exercising:

◆ **Set short-term goals.** A great way to motivate yourself is to create a definite, realistic plan for building endurance. If you are breathless after 10 minutes on the exercise bicycle, set a six-week goal of being able to bicycle for 20 minutes without panting. When you reach that goal, give yourself a small nonfood reward—perhaps a bubble bath, a new magazine, or a bouquet of flowers—for your accomplishment. Then, set a new goal immediately.

◆ **Set long-term goals.** Imagine a physical activity you have always wanted to do, but never seriously considered because you were so out of shape. Perhaps your fantasy is walking down the streets of an exotic city. Maybe you've always dreamed of mountain climbing. When you visualize yourself reaching this goal, you begin to get more in touch with your body and its possibilities.

◆ **Vary your routine.** Mixing and matching exercises, known as cross-training, helps you to work out different muscles while preventing you from feeling bored. A good approach is to try something you've never done before, such as the rowing or cross-country skiing machines, low-impact aerobics, or jazz dancing. You may also enjoy listening to music or watching television while you work out. If you are walking, change your route. Anything that makes your exercise routine more enjoyable and encourages you to stick with it is fine.

◆ **Use your Weight Control Journal.** Get in the habit of making regular entries. By recording the exercises you do, you can monitor your improving fitness level over time. When you look back on your records, it will be extremely satisfying to notice how much you've accomplished and how much stronger you are getting.

◆ **Plan ahead.** Decide what exercises you will be doing over at least the next two weeks and then follow your plan. Make sure your workout keeps pace with your fitness level.

◆ **Dress comfortably.** This may seem insignificant to you, but feeling comfortable is very impo﹒tant. Wear loose-fitting clothes—sweatpants and a T-shirt work well for many people—and make sure your shoes are appropriate.

◆ **Find a companion.** Exercising with a friend, or with a small group of people at a similar level, can be an excellent way to stay in the exercise habit.

◆ **Don't stop now.** It is easy to lose the conditioning you have worked so hard to achieve. If you stop your physical activities for as little as a month or two, you will quickly return to the fitness level from before you started exercising.

RULES FOR EXERCISE

Regardless of your specific approach to a well-conditioned body, the same basic rules apply:

◆ **Get a full medical checkup.** If you have any medical problems, or are over the age of 40, please consult your doctor before beginning the Getting Healthy exercise program. Almost everyone can custom-tailor my approach to their own fitness level, but it is smart to make sure you have no special restrictions.

◆ **Warm up properly.** The best approach is to begin with five minutes of gentle movement, followed by five minutes of gentle stretching, to increase the flow of blood through your body and to start your muscles working. Gentle movement might mean using exercise equipment on the lowest settings, walking slowly, or doing a light dance routine. When you have warmed up your muscles sufficiently, do some of the stretching exercises described in the next chapter.

◆ **Don't push too hard.** If you become dizzy, lightheaded, or short of breath, stop what you are doing and reduce the intensity of your exercise. Exercise should be rigorous, not painful. Save the more strenuous activities, such as jogging or weight lifting, until you are accustomed to regular physical activity.

◆ **Learn the rules.** Exercising properly, especially when you are using weights or machines, is important to avoid injury and to get the maximum benefit from your workout. You may want to work with an experienced friend or ask a professional trainer to evaluate your technique. It may also help to exercise in front of a mirror.

◆ **Cool down properly.** A few minutes of slow exercise or a few stretches at the end of your workout gives your body a chance to ease back to its relaxed state. A good cool-down also helps you avoid some of the muscle tightening and soreness that can accompany exercise.

THE OVERLOAD PRINCIPLE

In order to maintain a weight loss of more than 10 percent, you may have to overload your muscles by pushing them a little harder than they want to go. But I do mean just a little. You'll improve most, with the least risk of injury, if you push just slightly beyond your current ability. Your workout should feel hard, but not very hard.

Overloading means different things to different people. To someone who runs four miles a day, it may mean adding a fifth mile. But to someone who has been completely sedentary, it may mean nothing more than walking around the room while commercials are on television. That's fine. Take it slow and easy, and you'll be surprised at how much stronger you get, and how quickly.

As you continue to exercise, your overload has to keep pace with your conditioning. For example, when you reach the point where you can walk one half-hour a day easily, then you have to walk 35 minutes to build more muscle strength.

There are three ways to overload:

❖ Increase the frequency of your activity.

❖ Increase the duration of your activity.

❖ Increase the intensity of your activity.

The larger the weight loss you are trying to maintain, the more exercise you will need.

Frequency

Frequency is how often you do an exercise. If your current level of fitness results from walking around the block two or three times a week, you can improve by walking around the block four or five times a week. If you currently do push-ups twice a week, add an extra day to your routine.

Duration

Duration refers to the length of time you are currently exercising. You should increase the duration of activity by no more than 20 percent per week. If you have been walking 15 minutes a day, increase your walking time to 18 minutes next week and to 21 or 22 minutes the week after that. If you are using the walking program presented in the next chapter, increase your mileage by no more than one-half mile a week.

Intensity

Intensity is a measure of how hard you exercise. The trick is to work your muscles enough to strengthen them without overdoing it and risking injury. Exercising more intensively—for example, by picking up the pace of your walk—allows you to get the same workout in less time. You should increase the duration and frequency of your exercise first. Wait until you have established a steady exercise routine, which may take as long as 12 weeks, before you increase the intensity of your exercise.

16

DESIGNING YOUR OWN EXERCISE PROGRAM

As you have probably come to expect, the Getting Healthy exercise plan leaves plenty of room for individual decision making. I urge you to experiment with different kinds of exercise and to design a program that works for you. I don't expect everyone to work equally hard or long, but if you are serious about weight control, you can't be a couch potato.

If your life is already overloaded with commitments, even the modest requirements of my program may seem time-consuming. However, many people discover that they are so much more alert and efficient when they begin to exercise regularly that they eventually decide they can't afford not to exercise. You owe it to yourself, and to your commitment to weight control and a healthy life, to carve out the time for a modest workout.

If you experiment with different exercise regimens, you won't find it difficult to develop a program that works best for you, fits your schedule, and allows you to enjoy yourself, all at the same time. The mix of aerobic and resistance exercises presented in this chapter is flexible, easy to follow, and designed to help you become more physically fit. Remember, I've got only one immutable rule: *Exercise regularly.*

How Fit Are You?

By calculating a fitness baseline, you can enter my exercise program at the right level. This tool also helps you set goals and measure your progress.

The measured mile is one of the best ways to determine baseline fitness. Simply measure out a level one-mile route and walk it. Walk slightly faster than your usual stroll, but don't try for too speedy a pace. Use the second hand on your watch to determine how long it takes to complete the distance. The result is your fitness baseline, measured in minutes.

ONE-MILE TIMED WALK

Men	Women	Aerobic Condition
13:12 and under	14:40 and under	Excellent
13:13 to 14:42	14:41 to 16:08	Very Good
14:43 to 16:13	16:09 to 17:36	High Average
16:14 to 17:44	17:37 to 19:04	Low Average
17:45 to 19:23	19:05 to 20:31	Fair
19:24 and above	20:32 and above	Poor

Make an entry in your exercise log to show how long it took you to walk a mile. You will use that marker to determine your entry point into my walking program. As you become more fit, do the one-mile timed walk again from time to time to see how you are improving.

In general, you should underestimate your strength and endurance when you first start to exercise. It is much better to begin slowly than to risk injuring yourself because your stamina was not as great as you thought. If you have been fairly sedentary, it is smart to exercise just two or three times a week at first, although you will eventually have to build up to at least four days a week in order to reap the greatest possible weight control benefits.

THE BORG SCALE: HOW HARD SHOULD YOU EXERCISE?

The Borg scale was developed in the 1950s as a research tool to measure exertion in heart patients. This simple device helps you measure your own perception of how hard you are working out. For example, if you have been totally inactive, you may rank a short walk as "hard" (15 on the Borg scale) whereas you may perceive it as "very light" (9 on the Borg scale) if you are in good shape.

Using this scale of 6 to 20, indicate how you feel after doing a certain amount of exercise. Asking yourself these questions might help pinpoint the answer:

❖ How hard does this work feel?

❖ Am I breathing heavily?

❖ Am I perspiring?

❖ How do I feel after I am done?

THE BORG SCALE OF PERCEIVED EXERTION

6	
7	VERY, VERY LIGHT
8	
9	VERY LIGHT
10	
11	FAIRLY LIGHT
12	
13	SOMEWHAT HARD

14	
15	HARD
16	
17	VERY HARD
18	
19	VERY, VERY HARD
20	

A good, healthy aerobic workout should be done at the 13 or 14 level, with warm-ups and cooldowns in the 7 to 11 range. Resistance exercises should be less strenuous—aim for a Borg exertion level of 8 to 12. These levels allow your body to burn calories from fat most efficiently. Aerobic exercises above 15 are too hard and not necessary. In general, maximum weight control benefits are achieved by working at a hard, steady pace.

This scale is a great way to measure your improvement. As your strength builds, you will have to increase the intensity, frequency, or duration of your exercise to attain the same level of exertion. What made you feel highly fatigued three months ago may not feel like much at all now. By helping you monitor your own improving fitness level, instead of forcing you to measure up to someone else's standards, the Borg scale allows you to compete against the only person who matters here—you.

THE AEROBICS PROGRAM

During the first few weeks that you use the Getting Healthy approach to exercise, I suggest that you focus on building your aerobic capacity. Most people who have been sedentary find it easiest to begin with a walking program, but you may prefer some other form of aerobics, such as the bicycle, treadmill, or rowing machine. Whatever your preference, the goal is to exercise aerobically at least 20 minutes a day and no less often than every other day.

Stretching for Aerobic Exercises

Every aerobic workout should include some gentle stretching. To prevent the injury that can result from stretching cold muscles, start your body moving very gradually. Swinging your arms at your sides or taking a short walk are good pre-warm-ups.

Use the diagrams to guide you in a series of gentle muscle stretches, going as far as you can until you feel some mild resistance. Don't push yourself to the point of discomfort and never bounce. Hold each stretch for 30 seconds, repeat, and then move on to the next stretch. You don't need to use every stretch every time you exercise, but you should vary the stretches you do to help all parts of your body get limber. Stretch at least 5 minutes before walking.

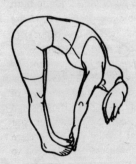

Standing Hamstring

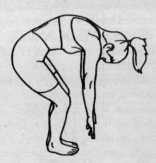

Standing Bent-Knee Hamstring

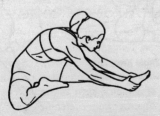

Seated One-Leg Hamstring

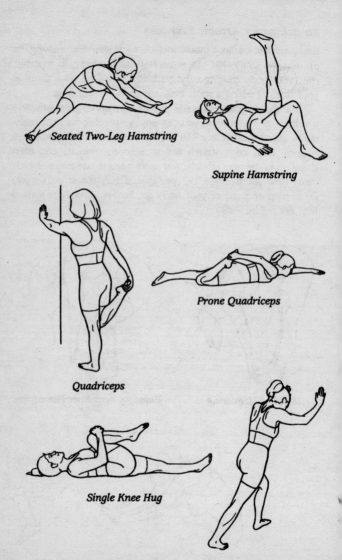

Seated Two-Leg Hamstring

Supine Hamstring

Quadriceps

Prone Quadriceps

Single Knee Hug

Calf

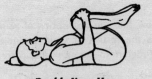

Double Knee Hug

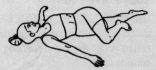

Knee Crossover

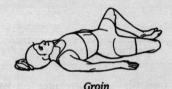

Groin

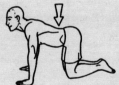

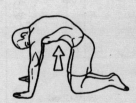

Back-Arch Stretch

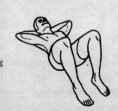

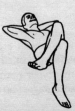

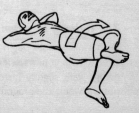

Lower-Torso Stretch

Your Entry Point

Using the Entry-Point Chart below, find the description of your aerobic condition that matches the results of your one-mile timed walk. Begin the Walking Program in the week that corresponds to that fitness level.

If you were unable to walk a full mile, start the program in the week with the number of minutes that you were able to walk. (For example, if you were able to walk for ten minutes, start at week three.)

ENTRY-POINT CHART

Results of One-Mile Timed Walk	Men Enter At Week	Women Enter At Week
Poor	4 to 6	3 to 5
Fair	5 to 7	4 to 6
Low Average	6 to 8	5 to 7
High Average	8 to 10	7 to 9
Very Good	10 to 12	9 to 11
Excellent	12	11

The Walking Program

Each walk should begin and end with a 5-minute, slow-paced stroll to help your muscles perform most efficiently. Once you get going, walk slightly faster than your normal pace. With every passing week, the program encourages you to walk a little farther.

Week Number	Warm-Up	Distance	Cooldown
1	5 minutes slow	5 minutes brisk	5 minutes slow
2	5 minutes slow	7 minutes brisk	5 minutes slow
3	5 minutes slow	9 minutes brisk	5 minutes slow
4	5 minutes slow	11 minutes brisk	5 minutes slow
5	5 minutes slow	13 minutes brisk	5 minutes slow
6	5 minutes slow	15 minutes brisk	5 minutes slow
7	5 minutes slow	18 minutes brisk	5 minutes slow
8	5 minutes slow	20 minutes brisk	5 minutes slow
9	5 minutes slow	23 minutes brisk	5 minutes slow
10	5 minutes slow	26 minutes brisk	5 minutes slow
11	5 minutes slow	28 minutes brisk	5 minutes slow
12	5 minutes slow	30 minutes brisk (approximately 1.5 to 2 miles)	5 minutes slow
13	5 minutes slow	33 minutes brisk	5 minutes slow

(continued)

Week Number	Warm-Up	Distance	Cooldown
14	5 minutes slow	36 minutes brisk	5 minutes slow
15	5 minutes slow	40 minutes brisk	5 minutes slow
16	5 minutes slow	45 minutes brisk (approximately 3 miles)	5 minutes slow

As a rule of thumb, you are walking fairly slowly if it takes you more than 18 minutes to walk a mile. A briskly walked mile takes between 14 and 17 minutes. Anything less than that is a high-intensity pace.

Increasing Intensity

After you have been walking for at least 12 weeks, you can increase the intensity of your aerobic workout to save time while building strength. One of the best ways is with interval training in which you work harder or faster for a short period of time and then slow down to catch your breath. For example, you can add a one-minute jog to every five minutes of walking. Exercise physiologists say there are important conditioning benefits to short bursts of higher-intensity exercise.

Here are some other ways that I recommend for increasing the intensity of your aerobic exercise:

❖ Walk up and down hills.

❖ Quicken your pace.

❖ Swing your arms fully as you walk.

THE RESISTANCE EXERCISE PROGRAM

Resistance exercises are less familiar to many Americans than the more popular aerobic exercises, such as jogging, dancing, and bicycle riding, but they are very important to weight control. Resistance training does not have to involve special equipment, but it may feel quite tiring at first. There is an art to building up your strength safely and gradually.

Stretching for Resistance Exercises

When you are ready to do resistance exercises, some new stretches focused on the upper body should be added to your routine. As with the aerobic stretches, you should stretch your muscles gently until you feel some mild tension. Don't push past that point or you may injure yourself. Hold each stretch for thirty seconds, repeat, and move on. Stretch for at least five minutes and vary the combinations that you use to loosen up all parts of your body.

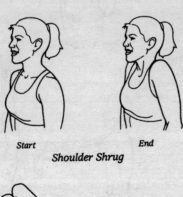

Start   **End**

Shoulder Shrug

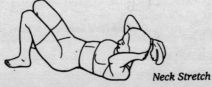

Neck Stretch

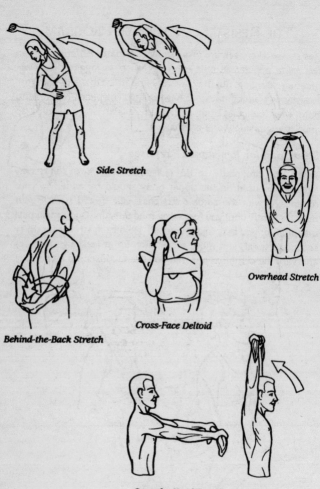

Side Stretch

Overhead Stretch

Behind-the-Back Stretch

Cross-Face Deltoid

Over-the-Head Stretch with Towel

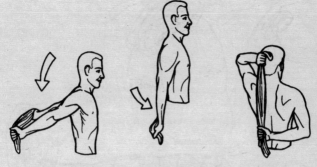

Behind-the-Back Stretch with Towel

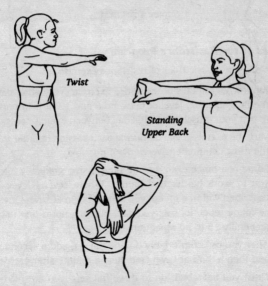

Twist

*Standing
Upper Back*

Behind-the-Head Triceps

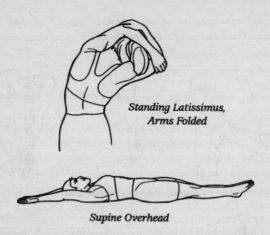

Standing Latissimus,
Arms Folded

Supine Overhead

Rules of the Resistance Program

Here are some basic rules of resistance exercise:

❖ Aim for 20 minutes of resistance exercise every other day at the Borg exertion level of between 8 and 12. It is important to rest your muscles for a full day between exercise sessions.

❖ Vary the exercises you do during each session in order to get the most comprehensive workout possible.

❖ Some resistance exercises are progressive, gradually forcing you to work harder and harder. Where several levels are described within a group, you should begin at Level One. Do as many repetitions as you can, building up to one full set (generally 15 to 20 repetitions).

❖ After you can comfortably do one full set, add a second set, and then a third at Level One. Rest a minute after each set.

❖ Once you have built up to three full sets, you are ready to move to a higher level within each group, if that option is provided. Ease into this by doing one set at Level Two, followed by two sets at the old level. Gradually replace the old exercise with the new one until you're doing three full sets at

Level Two. Continue this process until you build up to three sets at the highest level of each group.

❖ Try all of the rubber-band and weight exercises described here, because they strengthen different parts of the body. As you build muscle, increase the number of sets you do, up to a maximum of five. Add no more than one new set per group every one to two weeks.

❖ Remember the Overload Principle: Keep going a little past your comfort zone to gain maximum benefit. The last repetition of each exercise should feel as though you have reached your maximum capacity and should cause a slight muscle burning.

❖ Add simple, light weights to increase the intensity of your resistance exercises. You can use simple household items— such as a liter bottle of water or a can of food—or you can purchase an inexpensive set of weights at a local sporting goods store.

RESISTANCE EXERCISE GROUPS

Group I: Abdominals

Abdominal exercises tone and strengthen the stomach area.

Level One: Floor Crunches

One set = 15 to 20 repetitions

Lie on your back with your feet on the floor and your knees slightly bent. Your hands should rest at your sides.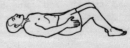

Raise your head and shoulders up so that your back comes off the floor. Your hands should reach toward your knees. Hold this position for 3 seconds and return to the floor.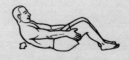

After you have built up to three sets of floor crunches, try these slightly more difficult variations:

Floor Crunch II Cross your arms in front of you and place your hands on your shoulders as you rise from the floor.

Floor Crunch III The hardest floor crunch requires you to place your hands beside or behind your head. Don't pull your head up—just rest your hands in this position as you rise from the floor.

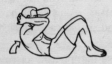

Level Two: Curl Crunches

One set = 15 to 20 repetitions

Lie on your back with your feet on the floor and your knees slightly bent. Place your hands behind your head with your elbows bent.

Raise your head and shoulders up so that your back comes off the floor. Bring your elbows in closer to your head. Hold this position for 3 seconds and return to the floor.

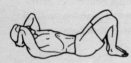

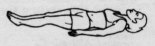

Level Three: Knee-Ups

One set = 15 to 20 repetitions

Lie on your back, with your hands just under your buttocks, palms down. Bring your knees slowly up to your chest, hold for 3 seconds, and come back down slowly.

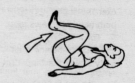

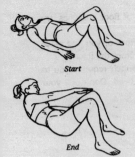

Start

End

Level Four: Cross Twists

One set = 10 repetitions on each side

Lie flat on the floor, with your arms stretched out by your sides and your knees bent. Raise your back and shoulders up and reach across your body, trying to touch your left knee with your right hand, then lie back down again.

Repeat 10 times, then reverse the exercise, touching the right knee with your left hand 10 times more.

For a slightly more difficult exercise, place your hands behind your head. Bring your elbows around slowly, again reaching for the opposite knee.

Level Five: Flat Cross Twists

One set = 10 repetitions on each side

The flat cross twist is similar to the cross twist except that your legs are straight. Lie flat on the floor, with your arms stretched out by your sides. Raise your back and shoulders up and reach across your body, trying to touch your left knee with both hands, then lie back down again.

Repeat 10 times, then reverse the exercise, touching the right knee with both hands 10 times more.

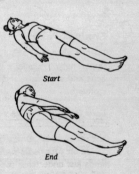

Start

End

For a slightly more difficult variation of this exercise, place your hands behind your head. Bring your elbow across your body slowly, reaching for the opposite knee.

Level Six: Pelvic Tilt

One set = 15 to 20 rep-
etitions

Lie on your back
with your knees raised
and your hands behind
your head. Thrust your
back and buttocks
upward, keeping your
feet flat on the floor.
Hold for several seconds
and return to the floor.

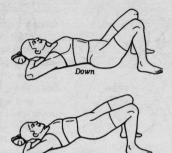

Group II: Pushes

Pushes are very helpful to the
upper body, especially the triceps and shoulders, and to the
stomach.

Level One: Wall Pushes

One set = 15 to 20 repetitions

Stand with your elbows
bent, your feet flat on the floor,
and your hands against a wall.
Incline your body slightly
inward. Keeping your back
straight, push away from the
wall until your elbows are
straight. Your arms should be
slightly lower than shoulder
height.

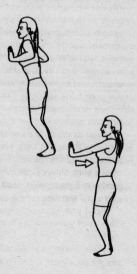

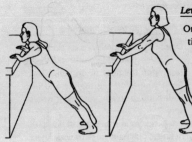

Level Two: Counter Pushes

One set = 15 to 20 repetitions

With your feet flat on the floor and your elbows slightly bent, place your hands on a kitchen counter. Keep your back straight as you incline slightly down toward the counter, then push away.

Level Three: Knee Pushes

One set = 15 to 20 repetitions

Kneel down with your knees touching the floor, your palms down, elbows bent, and hands placed shoulder-width apart. Slowly push yourself up with your hands until your arms are stretched out full, leaving your knees touching the floor.

Make sure your back remains straight throughout the exercise.

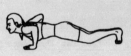

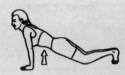

Level Four: Push-Ups

One set = 15 to 20 repetitions

Stretch out on your stomach, with your legs fully extended, your hands placed shoulder-width apart, and your elbows bent. Slowly push up with your hands until your weight rests only on your arms and toes.

Bend your elbows and move back down until you are about 1 inch from the floor.

Make sure your back remains straight throughout the exercise.

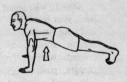

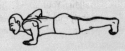

Group III: Hips and Buttocks

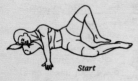

Start

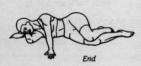

End

Level One: External Rotations

One set = 10 repetitions on each side

Lie on your side, with your head resting on the floor or on your hand. Bend your lower leg slightly and use your hand to steady yourself if necessary.

Bend your top knee at least 90 degrees, pulling it close to your chest. Rotate the top knee toward the floor and back. Make sure the knee rotates and your heel stays stationary. After 10 repetitions, reverse sides.

Level Two: Three-Angle Leg Raises

One set = 10 repetitions with each leg

Lie on your side, with your head resting on the floor or on your hand. Raise your leg to a 90-degree angle, then lower it.

Then, extend the leg out to a 75-degree angle, then lower it.

Repeat at a 45-degree angle.

After 10 repetitions, do the same with the opposite leg.

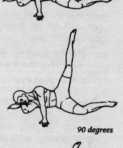

90 degrees

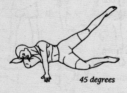

45 degrees

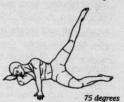

75 degrees

Group IV: Back

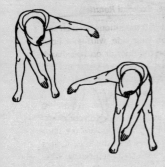

Windmill

One set = 15 to 20 repetitions

Stand up straight, feet shoulder-length apart. With knees slightly bent, lean down, bringing your right hand as close to the toes of your left foot as possible.

Stand back up straight and then bend again, bringing your left hand as far toward the toes of your right foot as possible.

Group V: Rubber-Band Exercises

An extra-strong and extra-large rubber band can be purchased inexpensively at hospital supply or sporting goods stores. These exercises help strengthen all parts of the upper body—the chest, arms, back, and shoulders. As you gain strength, you can use bands with increasing levels of resistance.

Butterfly

One set = 15 to 20 repetitions

Wrap the rubber band around your hands. Extend your arms in front of your body at shoulder height. Pull the ends of the bands, spreading your arms out to your side. Pinch your shoulder blades together as you stretch out your arms and hold for a few seconds. Slowly return to the starting position.

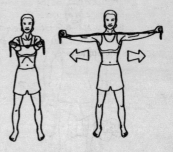

Bow and Arrow

One set = 15 to 20 repetitions

Wrap one end of the rubber band around each hand. Extend your arms straight out in front of your body.

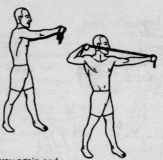

Keeping one arm stationary in front of you, pull back the band with the other hand and hold for 3 seconds.

Bring both arms in front of you again and reverse arms.

Standing Row

One set = 15 to 20 repetitions

Stand with your feet shoulder-width apart. Step on the band in the middle. Hold the ends in your hands; for a better grip, wrap them around your hands.

Start with both arms extended in front of you, then pull both arms up simultaneously and hold for a few seconds.

Lower your hands back to their resting position.

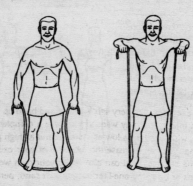

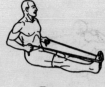

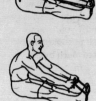

Seated Cable Row

One set = 15 to 20 repetitions

Sit upright on the floor with your feet together. Wrap the band around the bottom of your feet and hold one end with each hand.

Extend your arms in front of you and pull back on the band with both arms simultaneously. Pinch your shoulder blades together as you pull.

Hold for several seconds and slowly return your hands to a resting position.

Biceps Curl

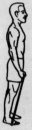

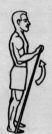

One set = 10 repetitions with each arm

Stand on one end of the band and wrap the other end around one hand. Start with your arm down at your side. Bend your elbow, keeping your wrist straight, and pull the band up toward your body. Hold for several seconds, then uncurl your arm until you return to your original position. After 10 repetitions, switch to the other arm.

Group VI: Weights

Begin weight exercises with very light weights and build up gradually to avoid injury. You may want to purchase a complete set of dumbbells, with weights as low as 1 pound and as high as 15 pounds, so that you can increase the intensity of your exercise as you become stronger. You can also make your own weights with soup cans or by filling one-liter bottles with sand, pennies, or water.

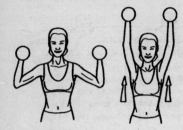

Overhead Press

One set = 15 to 20 repetitions

Stand with your elbows bent, holding the weights up. Extend your arms straight up. If possible, allow your hands to touch briefly.

Return arms slowly to your starting position.

Lateral Raise

One set = 15 to 20 repetitions

Start with your hands hanging down at your sides, holding the weights. With elbows locked and palms facing the floor, lift both arms simultaneously away from your sides until they are at shoulder height.

Return arms slowly to your starting position.

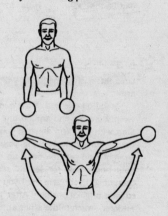

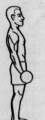

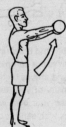

Front Raise

One set = 15 to 20 repetitions

Start with your arms hanging down at your sides, holding the weights. With elbows locked and palms facing your body, lift both arms together in front of you until they reach shoulder height.

Return arms slowly to your starting position.

Triceps Kickbacks

One set = 15 to 20 repetitions

Bend your knees slightly. Bend your elbows, holding the weights so that your upper arm is parallel to the floor and your forearm is perpendicular to the floor. Extend your arms straight back behind your body.

Return arms slowly to your starting position.

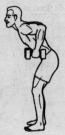
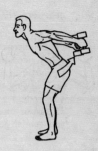

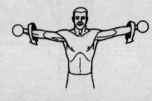

Arm Circles

One set = 10 repetitions in each direction

Extend your arms straight out from your sides, holding the weight palms down.

Slowly rotate your arms in small circles, first clockwise ten times, then counterclockwise ten times.

Punches

One set = 15 to 20 repetitions

With palms facing each other, extend your right arm straight out in front of you in slow and deliberate motion. Bend at the elbow and pull the arm back in. Then, extend the left arm out slowly and deliberately and pull it back in.

Alternate between the right and left arms.

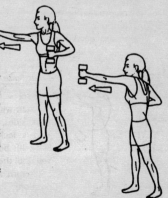

Triceps Overhead Extension

One set = 15 to 20 repetitions

Bend your elbows and hold the weights behind your head, with your palms facing forward. Slowly straighten your elbows and extend the weights straight
up following the line of
your body. .

Return arms slowly to
your starting position.

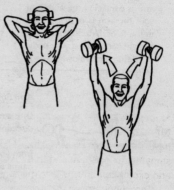

A FINAL WORD

———— ❖ ————

Congratulations! I'm really pleased by how far you've come. No matter how much weight you have lost by now, I think you have shown impressive fortitude and stick-to-it-iveness just by studying my program and thinking about the dietary, behavioral, and exercise programs that might work for you.

Throughout this book, I've tried to be straightforward about the challenges you may face. Losing excess weight is never an easy job, but I'm sure it hasn't been easy dealing with a weight problem for much of your life either. Weight control is a learned skill, something that becomes easier with practice. People do succeed; I see it happen all the time. Once you learn to play by the rules—and mine are structured with a great deal of flexibility—you will have a foundation of knowledge upon which to build. Although the struggle to maintain weight takes a lifetime, the rewards of good health make it all worthwhile.

Fortunately, this is a period of tremendous creative ferment in my field. The discovery of the *ob* gene and the leptin hormone and new insights about metabolism and brain chemistry reinforce the theory that obesity is a medical condition, which may help physicians treat people with weight problems in new ways. In my own practice, I tell my patients there are always other options we can try. Although faddish diets don't work, some people are successful on a 1,200-calorie diet, even if the guidelines I've given you would allow a higher caloric intake. Where appropriate, I sometimes complement my program of diet, exercise, and behavioral changes with medications. Under some circumstances, surgery can also be considered.

The drugs in common use today—phentermine and fenfluramine—work in two main ways and are used alone or in combination with each other:

1. They suppress your appetite so that you eat less.
2. They may stimulate your metabolism so that you burn more calories.

Unfortunately, these drugs only work in about 50% of the population and can have side effects. Also, they haven't been fully studied for long-term use. Although most people are able to tolerate phentermine and fenfluramine, it is important that the user be monitored regularly by the physician who prescribes them.

Researchers are also studying drugs that may prevent your body from absorbing calories and those that may reduce insulin resistance. And, of course, the prospect of leptin therapy to alter the body's fat-regulating mechanism is enormously promising. If you have followed the Getting Healthy principles carefully, tried both Menu Plan I and Menu Plan II, and have not achieved a weight loss averaging a pound every other week after four months, you may want to discuss medication with your doctor. But remember, medication may give you a boost but it won't substitute for the rest of my program.

Surgery is only appropriate for individuals who have been at more than twice their desired body weight for at least five years and have failed all other treatments. Two techniques are in use:

1. Gastric bypass surgery, which reroutes some of the intestine so that your body cannot absorb excess calories. If you overeat, you will suffer from severe diarrhea.

2. Stomach stapling, which reduces the size of your stomach so that you feel very full, very quickly. You are likely to vomit any excess food you consume.

Surgery has both short-term and long-term complications, but its benefits may outweigh its risks for some seriously overweight people, especially those who are already suffering from health problems. You will need extensive medical follow-up and education in new ways of eating and exercising.

I expect these methods and other pharmacological and surgical techniques will be refined in coming years, but I doubt they will ever eliminate the relevance of the three-point Getting Healthy program. Nor will they erase the damaging and ignorant stereotypes that linger about fat people. Chances are that you have had firsthand experience with some of them. The national obsession with thinness has driven many with weight problems into the arms of quacks and quick-buck hucksters who offer outlandish treatments and promise easy cures. In many circles, people who are overweight are still being blamed for their bodies, rather than helped to change them.

An enormous amount of work needs to be done to eliminate stereotypes and to educate people about the realities of obesity and weight control. You can play an important role in this process. Let other people know that good health, not beauty, is the objective of a sound weight-loss program. Talk about your own experiences. Get involved with consumer groups trying to spread the word. Encourage your medical providers to learn more about nutrition and to emphasize preventive approaches to weight control. Be a friend to someone who is still struggling through Dark Age attitudes.

In short, become involved. As you fight your own battles, you will be sending a message that may help others lead better, healthier lives. I'm proud to be part of that effort, and I'd be happy to have you join me.

RESOURCES

———————— ❖ ————————

BOOKS AND RECIPE SOURCES

I'm delighted to see so many new books and magazines being published that emphasize sound nutrition and healthy eating. There are also a number of excellent sources on some of the political and psychological issues that are often associated with weight problems. Although I'm including a list of my favorite books and magazines, I recommend that you browse through your local bookstore or library to find other good resources.

Nutrition Book (Bantam, 1988)
Good Food Book (Bantam, 1987)
by Jane Brody
   This *New York Times* columnist takes a knowledgeable, common-sense approach that is useful both for the average consumer and for the health-care professional.

Great Good Food (Crown, 1993)
by Julee Rosso
Gourmet recipes with a healthy bent.

Provençal Light (Bantam, 1994)
Mediterranean Light (Bantam, 1989)
by Martha Rose Shulman
Recipes that emphasize the Mediterranean approach to eating—plenty of olive oil, grains, and yogurt, and not too much meat.

In the Kitchen with Rosie (Knopf, 1994)
by Rosie Daley
The bestselling book featuring recipes that helped Oprah Winfrey shed all those extra pounds.

The Joy of Snacks (Chronimed, 1991)
by Nancy Cooper
Snacks featuring low-calorie, low-fat, and low-sugar goodies. Many of the snacks are great for children.

Weight Watchers 365-Day Menu Cookbook (Plume, 1993)
Weight Watchers Favorite Recipes (Plume, 1988)
Weight Watchers New International Cookbook (Plume, 1985)
Excellent recipe collections that show inviting ways to present food and food exchanges that work.

Cooking Lite
Eating Well
Monthly magazines, available at many newsstands, filled with nutritional and tasty low-fat recipes. The editors of both magazines are registered dietitians.

Breaking Free from Compulsive Overeating (Plume, 1993)
When Food Is Love (Plume, 1992)
by Geneen Roth
This author is particularly good at helping people untangle the complex food/emotion knot.

Wherever You Go, There You Are (Hyperion, 1994)
Full Catastrophe Living: Using the Wisdom of Your Body and Mind to Face Stress, Pain and Illness (Delta, 1991)
by Jonathan Kabot Zim

Both books provide excellent guides to stress reduction and the art of coping.

Fat Is a Feminist Issue (Berkley, 1994)
by Susie Orbach

Political and psychological insights about what it is like to be overweight. I recommend this book to both men and women.

Feeling Good: The New Mood Therapy (Avon, 1992)
The Feeling Good Handbook (New American Library/Dutton, 1990)
by David Burns

Excellent guides to depression, with important insights about self-image, including how overweight people think of themselves.

EXERCISE VIDEOTAPES

Most video stores carry a number of exercise videotapes that have been prepared with professional guidance. Using those listed below, or others, may give you the support to stick with an exercise program.

Jane Fonda's Complete Workout
Jane Fonda's Lower Body Solution
Jane Fonda's Lean Routine

Jane Fonda's videotapes include about 15 minutes on nutrition and a 50-minute workout.

Sweatin' to the Oldies
Richard Simmons

A classic exercise videotape with great music. My patients really enjoy this one.

OTHER WEIGHT CONTROL RESOURCES

The LEARN Program
The LEARN Education Center
1555 West Mockingbird Lane
Suite 203
Dallas, TX 75235
1-800-736-7323
    One of the most responsible weight-loss programs available is the LEARN Program for Weight Control (short for Lifestyle, Exercise, Attitudes, Relationships, and Nutrition). The LEARN Education Center has developed a very useful weight-loss manual, audiotapes, and other valuable resources.

Weight Watchers
1-800-651-6000
    This is the only commercial weight control program that I can recommend enthusiastically. It is practical, well focused, and provides credible information about menu planning and food exchanges. Call the toll-free number to find the Weight Watchers group nearest you.

Overeaters Anonymous
Box 44020
Rio Rancho, NM 87174
1-505-891-2664
    Overeaters Anonymous is a nationwide twelve-step rehabilitation program targeted at compulsive eaters. It helps many people with eating disorders to get into a group that can share and understand their problems in a way that noncompulsives never can. There are OA groups in many regions of the country. Check your local telephone book for the one nearest you or contact the national office for a referral.

American Dietetic Association
1-800-366-1655

This is the national credentialing association for registered dietitians, and it maintains referral lists for most regions of the country.

Exercise Resources

Finding a Personal Trainer
For a referral to a personal trainer in your area, visit your local gym and ask for a referral. Or you can call the Aerobics and Fitness Association of America at 1-800-983-2677.

Purchasing Weights and Rubber Bands
Most sporting goods stores will have a selection of the relatively inexpensive weights and rubber bands you will need to do your resistance exercises. A good mail-order source is Fitness Wholesale at 1-800-537-5512.

Audiotapes

Myths, Metaphors and Messages: The Magic of Hypno-Peripheral Processing

Available from: New Marketing
360 French Court
Teaneck, NJ 07666

Audiotapes by Dr. Lloyd Glauberman designed to help you address some of the subconscious issues that may play a role in weight control. Some of my patients confirm that these are a quantum leap beyond hypnosis and other subliminal tapes.

INDEX